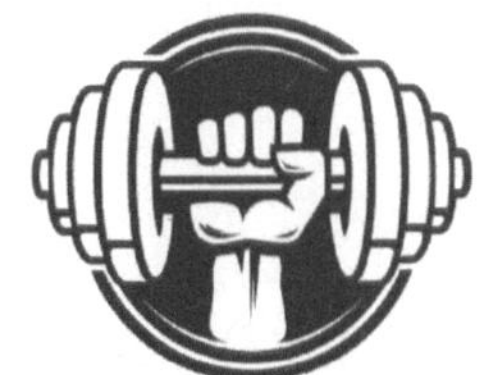

NAME:_____________

DATE:_____________

TIME START:_____________

TIME END:_____________

| WARM-UP | TIME | NOTES |
|---|---|---|
|  |  |  |
|  |  |  |
|  |  |  |
|  |  |  |

| EXERCISE: | SET 1 | | SET 2 | | SET 3 | | SET 4 | |
|---|---|---|---|---|---|---|---|---|
|  | REPS | WEIGHT | REPS | WEIGHT | REPS | WEIGHT | REPS | WEIGHT |
|  |  |  |  |  |  |  |  |  |
|  |  |  |  |  |  |  |  |  |
|  |  |  |  |  |  |  |  |  |
|  |  |  |  |  |  |  |  |  |
|  |  |  |  |  |  |  |  |  |
|  |  |  |  |  |  |  |  |  |
|  |  |  |  |  |  |  |  |  |
|  |  |  |  |  |  |  |  |  |
|  |  |  |  |  |  |  |  |  |
|  |  |  |  |  |  |  |  |  |
|  |  |  |  |  |  |  |  |  |
|  |  |  |  |  |  |  |  |  |

| CARDIO: | TIME | DISTANCE | PACE | HR |
|---|---|---|---|---|
|  |  |  |  |  |
|  |  |  |  |  |
|  |  |  |  |  |
|  |  |  |  |  |

| SUPPLEMENTS & VITAMINS | SERVINGS | QUANTITY |
|---|---|---|
|  |  |  |
|  |  |  |
|  |  |  |
|  |  |  |
|  |  |  |

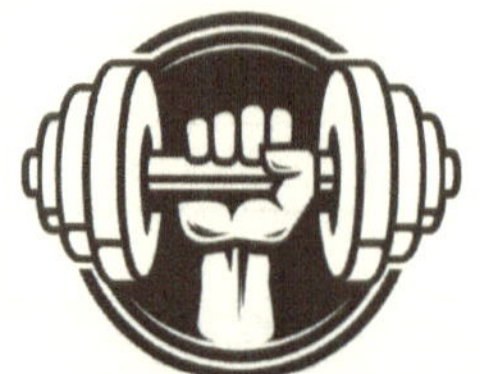

NAME:

DATE:

TIME START:

TIME END:

| WARM-UP | TIME | NOTES |
|---|---|---|
|  |  |  |
|  |  |  |
|  |  |  |
|  |  |  |

| EXERCISE: | SET 1 | | SET 2 | | SET 3 | | SET 4 | |
|---|---|---|---|---|---|---|---|---|
|  | REPS | WEIGHT | REPS | WEIGHT | REPS | WEIGHT | REPS | WEIGHT |
|  |  |  |  |  |  |  |  |  |
|  |  |  |  |  |  |  |  |  |
|  |  |  |  |  |  |  |  |  |
|  |  |  |  |  |  |  |  |  |
|  |  |  |  |  |  |  |  |  |
|  |  |  |  |  |  |  |  |  |
|  |  |  |  |  |  |  |  |  |
|  |  |  |  |  |  |  |  |  |
|  |  |  |  |  |  |  |  |  |
|  |  |  |  |  |  |  |  |  |
|  |  |  |  |  |  |  |  |  |
|  |  |  |  |  |  |  |  |  |

| CARDIO: | TIME | DISTANCE | PACE | HR |
|---|---|---|---|---|
|  |  |  |  |  |
|  |  |  |  |  |
|  |  |  |  |  |
|  |  |  |  |  |

| SUPPLEMENTS & VITAMINS | SERVINGS | QUANTITY |
|---|---|---|
|  |  |  |
|  |  |  |
|  |  |  |
|  |  |  |
|  |  |  |

NAME:_______________________

DATE:_______________________

TIME START:_______________________

TIME END:_______________________

| WARM-UP | TIME | NOTES |
|---|---|---|
|  |  |  |
|  |  |  |
|  |  |  |
|  |  |  |

| EXERCISE: | SET 1 | | SET 2 | | SET 3 | | SET 4 | |
|---|---|---|---|---|---|---|---|---|
|  | REPS | WEIGHT | REPS | WEIGHT | REPS | WEIGHT | REPS | WEIGHT |
|  |  |  |  |  |  |  |  |  |
|  |  |  |  |  |  |  |  |  |
|  |  |  |  |  |  |  |  |  |
|  |  |  |  |  |  |  |  |  |
|  |  |  |  |  |  |  |  |  |
|  |  |  |  |  |  |  |  |  |
|  |  |  |  |  |  |  |  |  |
|  |  |  |  |  |  |  |  |  |
|  |  |  |  |  |  |  |  |  |
|  |  |  |  |  |  |  |  |  |
|  |  |  |  |  |  |  |  |  |
|  |  |  |  |  |  |  |  |  |

| CARDIO: | TIME | DISTANCE | PACE | HR |
|---|---|---|---|---|
|  |  |  |  |  |
|  |  |  |  |  |
|  |  |  |  |  |
|  |  |  |  |  |

| SUPPLEMENTS & VITAMINS | SERVINGS | QUANTITY |
|---|---|---|
|  |  |  |
|  |  |  |
|  |  |  |
|  |  |  |
|  |  |  |

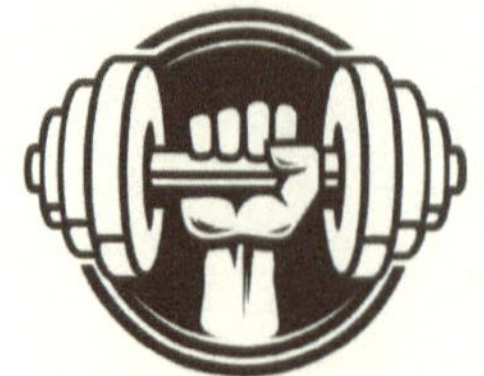

NAME:

DATE:

TIME START:

TIME END:

| WARM-UP | TIME | NOTES |
|---|---|---|
|  |  |  |
|  |  |  |
|  |  |  |
|  |  |  |

| EXERCISE: | SET 1 | | SET 2 | | SET 3 | | SET 4 | |
|---|---|---|---|---|---|---|---|---|
|  | REPS | WEIGHT | REPS | WEIGHT | REPS | WEIGHT | REPS | WEIGHT |
|  |  |  |  |  |  |  |  |  |
|  |  |  |  |  |  |  |  |  |
|  |  |  |  |  |  |  |  |  |
|  |  |  |  |  |  |  |  |  |
|  |  |  |  |  |  |  |  |  |
|  |  |  |  |  |  |  |  |  |
|  |  |  |  |  |  |  |  |  |
|  |  |  |  |  |  |  |  |  |
|  |  |  |  |  |  |  |  |  |
|  |  |  |  |  |  |  |  |  |
|  |  |  |  |  |  |  |  |  |
|  |  |  |  |  |  |  |  |  |

| CARDIO: | TIME | DISTANCE | PACE | HR |
|---|---|---|---|---|
|  |  |  |  |  |
|  |  |  |  |  |
|  |  |  |  |  |
|  |  |  |  |  |

| SUPPLEMENTS & VITAMINS | SERVINGS | QUANTITY |
|---|---|---|
|  |  |  |
|  |  |  |
|  |  |  |
|  |  |  |

| NAME: | |
| DATE: | |
| TIME START: | |
| TIME END: | |

| WARM-UP | TIME | NOTES |
|---|---|---|
| | | |
| | | |
| | | |
| | | |

| EXERCISE: | SET 1 | | SET 2 | | SET 3 | | SET 4 | |
|---|---|---|---|---|---|---|---|---|
| | REPS | WEIGHT | REPS | WEIGHT | REPS | WEIGHT | REPS | WEIGHT |
| | | | | | | | | |
| | | | | | | | | |
| | | | | | | | | |
| | | | | | | | | |
| | | | | | | | | |
| | | | | | | | | |
| | | | | | | | | |
| | | | | | | | | |
| | | | | | | | | |
| | | | | | | | | |
| | | | | | | | | |

| CARDIO: | TIME | DISTANCE | PACE | HR |
|---|---|---|---|---|
| | | | | |
| | | | | |
| | | | | |
| | | | | |

| SUPPLEMENTS & VITAMINS | SERVINGS | QUANTITY |
|---|---|---|
| | | |
| | | |
| | | |
| | | |
| | | |

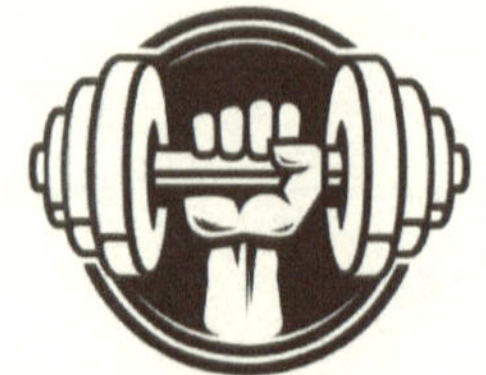

NAME:

DATE:

TIME START:

TIME END:

| WARM-UP | TIME | NOTES |
|---|---|---|
|  |  |  |
|  |  |  |
|  |  |  |
|  |  |  |

| EXERCISE: | SET 1 | | SET 2 | | SET 3 | | SET 4 | |
|---|---|---|---|---|---|---|---|---|
|  | REPS | WEIGHT | REPS | WEIGHT | REPS | WEIGHT | REPS | WEIGHT |
|  |  |  |  |  |  |  |  |  |
|  |  |  |  |  |  |  |  |  |
|  |  |  |  |  |  |  |  |  |
|  |  |  |  |  |  |  |  |  |
|  |  |  |  |  |  |  |  |  |
|  |  |  |  |  |  |  |  |  |
|  |  |  |  |  |  |  |  |  |
|  |  |  |  |  |  |  |  |  |
|  |  |  |  |  |  |  |  |  |
|  |  |  |  |  |  |  |  |  |
|  |  |  |  |  |  |  |  |  |

| CARDIO: | TIME | DISTANCE | PACE | HR |
|---|---|---|---|---|
|  |  |  |  |  |
|  |  |  |  |  |
|  |  |  |  |  |
|  |  |  |  |  |

| SUPPLEMENTS & VITAMINS | SERVINGS | QUANTITY |
|---|---|---|
|  |  |  |
|  |  |  |
|  |  |  |
|  |  |  |

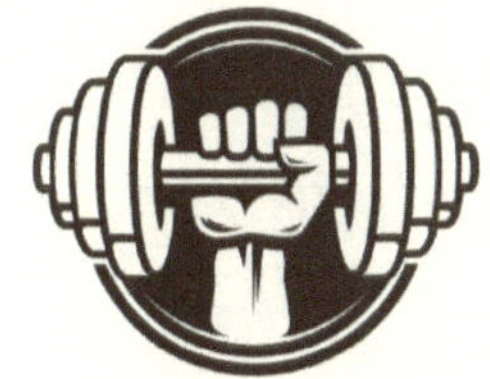



| WARM-UP | TIME | NOTES |
|---|---|---|
|  |  |  |
|  |  |  |
|  |  |  |
|  |  |  |

| EXERCISE: | SET 1 | | SET 2 | | SET 3 | | SET 4 | |
|---|---|---|---|---|---|---|---|---|
|  | REPS | WEIGHT | REPS | WEIGHT | REPS | WEIGHT | REPS | WEIGHT |
|  |  |  |  |  |  |  |  |  |
|  |  |  |  |  |  |  |  |  |
|  |  |  |  |  |  |  |  |  |
|  |  |  |  |  |  |  |  |  |
|  |  |  |  |  |  |  |  |  |
|  |  |  |  |  |  |  |  |  |
|  |  |  |  |  |  |  |  |  |
|  |  |  |  |  |  |  |  |  |
|  |  |  |  |  |  |  |  |  |

| CARDIO: | TIME | DISTANCE | PACE | HR |
|---|---|---|---|---|
|  |  |  |  |  |
|  |  |  |  |  |
|  |  |  |  |  |
|  |  |  |  |  |

| SUPPLEMENTS & VITAMINS | SERVINGS | QUANTITY |
|---|---|---|
|  |  |  |
|  |  |  |
|  |  |  |
|  |  |  |
|  |  |  |

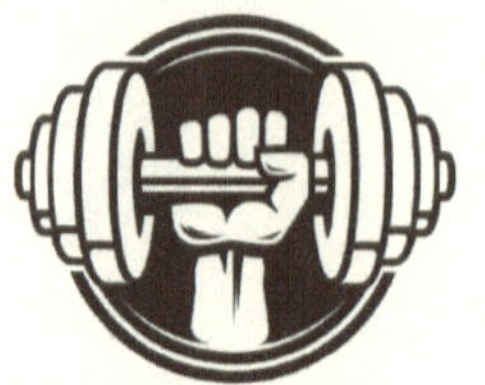

NAME:_______________________

DATE:_______________________

TIME START:_______________________

TIME END:_______________________

| WARM-UP | TIME | NOTES |
|---|---|---|
|  |  |  |
|  |  |  |
|  |  |  |

| EXERCISE: | SET 1 | | SET 2 | | SET 3 | | SET 4 | |
|---|---|---|---|---|---|---|---|---|
|  | REPS | WEIGHT | REPS | WEIGHT | REPS | WEIGHT | REPS | WEIGHT |
|  |  |  |  |  |  |  |  |  |
|  |  |  |  |  |  |  |  |  |
|  |  |  |  |  |  |  |  |  |
|  |  |  |  |  |  |  |  |  |
|  |  |  |  |  |  |  |  |  |
|  |  |  |  |  |  |  |  |  |
|  |  |  |  |  |  |  |  |  |
|  |  |  |  |  |  |  |  |  |
|  |  |  |  |  |  |  |  |  |
|  |  |  |  |  |  |  |  |  |
|  |  |  |  |  |  |  |  |  |

| CARDIO: | TIME | DISTANCE | PACE | HR |
|---|---|---|---|---|
|  |  |  |  |  |
|  |  |  |  |  |
|  |  |  |  |  |

| SUPPLEMENTS & VITAMINS | SERVINGS | QUANTITY |
|---|---|---|
|  |  |  |
|  |  |  |
|  |  |  |

NAME:_______________________________

DATE:_______________________________

TIME START:_______________________________

TIME END:_______________________________

| WARM-UP | TIME | NOTES |
| --- | --- | --- |
|  |  |  |
|  |  |  |
|  |  |  |
|  |  |  |

| EXERCISE: | SET 1 | | SET 2 | | SET 3 | | SET 4 | |
| --- | --- | --- | --- | --- | --- | --- | --- | --- |
|  | REPS | WEIGHT | REPS | WEIGHT | REPS | WEIGHT | REPS | WEIGHT |
|  |  |  |  |  |  |  |  |  |
|  |  |  |  |  |  |  |  |  |
|  |  |  |  |  |  |  |  |  |
|  |  |  |  |  |  |  |  |  |
|  |  |  |  |  |  |  |  |  |
|  |  |  |  |  |  |  |  |  |
|  |  |  |  |  |  |  |  |  |
|  |  |  |  |  |  |  |  |  |
|  |  |  |  |  |  |  |  |  |
|  |  |  |  |  |  |  |  |  |
|  |  |  |  |  |  |  |  |  |

| CARDIO: | TIME | DISTANCE | PACE | HR |
| --- | --- | --- | --- | --- |
|  |  |  |  |  |
|  |  |  |  |  |
|  |  |  |  |  |
|  |  |  |  |  |

| SUPPLEMENTS & VITAMINS | SERVINGS | QUANTITY |
| --- | --- | --- |
|  |  |  |
|  |  |  |
|  |  |  |
|  |  |  |
|  |  |  |

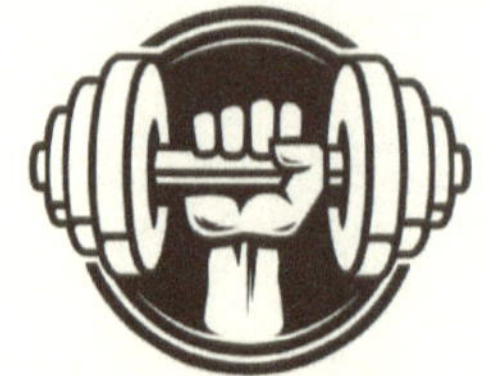

NAME:

DATE:

TIME START:

TIME END:

| WARM-UP | TIME | NOTES |
|---|---|---|
|  |  |  |
|  |  |  |
|  |  |  |
|  |  |  |

| EXERCISE: | SET 1 | | SET 2 | | SET 3 | | SET 4 | |
|---|---|---|---|---|---|---|---|---|
|  | REPS | WEIGHT | REPS | WEIGHT | REPS | WEIGHT | REPS | WEIGHT |
|  |  |  |  |  |  |  |  |  |
|  |  |  |  |  |  |  |  |  |
|  |  |  |  |  |  |  |  |  |
|  |  |  |  |  |  |  |  |  |
|  |  |  |  |  |  |  |  |  |
|  |  |  |  |  |  |  |  |  |
|  |  |  |  |  |  |  |  |  |
|  |  |  |  |  |  |  |  |  |
|  |  |  |  |  |  |  |  |  |
|  |  |  |  |  |  |  |  |  |
|  |  |  |  |  |  |  |  |  |
|  |  |  |  |  |  |  |  |  |

| CARDIO: | TIME | DISTANCE | PACE | HR |
|---|---|---|---|---|
|  |  |  |  |  |
|  |  |  |  |  |
|  |  |  |  |  |
|  |  |  |  |  |

| SUPPLEMENTS & VITAMINS | SERVINGS | QUANTITY |
|---|---|---|
|  |  |  |
|  |  |  |
|  |  |  |
|  |  |  |

NAME:_______________________

DATE:_______________________

TIME START:_______________________

TIME END:_______________________

| WARM-UP | TIME | NOTES |
|---------|------|-------|
|  |  |  |
|  |  |  |
|  |  |  |
|  |  |  |

| EXERCISE: | SET 1 | | SET 2 | | SET 3 | | SET 4 | |
|-----------|-------|--------|-------|--------|-------|--------|-------|--------|
|  | REPS | WEIGHT | REPS | WEIGHT | REPS | WEIGHT | REPS | WEIGHT |
|  |  |  |  |  |  |  |  |  |
|  |  |  |  |  |  |  |  |  |
|  |  |  |  |  |  |  |  |  |
|  |  |  |  |  |  |  |  |  |
|  |  |  |  |  |  |  |  |  |
|  |  |  |  |  |  |  |  |  |
|  |  |  |  |  |  |  |  |  |
|  |  |  |  |  |  |  |  |  |
|  |  |  |  |  |  |  |  |  |
|  |  |  |  |  |  |  |  |  |
|  |  |  |  |  |  |  |  |  |
|  |  |  |  |  |  |  |  |  |

| CARDIO: | TIME | DISTANCE | PACE | HR |
|---------|------|----------|------|----|
|  |  |  |  |  |
|  |  |  |  |  |
|  |  |  |  |  |
|  |  |  |  |  |

| SUPPLEMENTS & VITAMINS | SERVINGS | QUANTITY |
|------------------------|----------|----------|
|  |  |  |
|  |  |  |
|  |  |  |
|  |  |  |
|  |  |  |

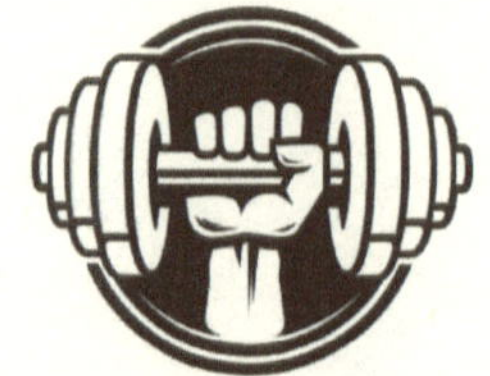

NAME:

DATE:

TIME START:

TIME END:

| WARM-UP | TIME | NOTES |
|---------|------|-------|
|  |  |  |
|  |  |  |
|  |  |  |
|  |  |  |

| EXERCISE: | SET 1 | | SET 2 | | SET 3 | | SET 4 | |
|-----------|-------|--------|-------|--------|-------|--------|-------|--------|
|  | REPS | WEIGHT | REPS | WEIGHT | REPS | WEIGHT | REPS | WEIGHT |
|  |  |  |  |  |  |  |  |  |
|  |  |  |  |  |  |  |  |  |
|  |  |  |  |  |  |  |  |  |
|  |  |  |  |  |  |  |  |  |
|  |  |  |  |  |  |  |  |  |
|  |  |  |  |  |  |  |  |  |
|  |  |  |  |  |  |  |  |  |
|  |  |  |  |  |  |  |  |  |
|  |  |  |  |  |  |  |  |  |
|  |  |  |  |  |  |  |  |  |
|  |  |  |  |  |  |  |  |  |
|  |  |  |  |  |  |  |  |  |

| CARDIO: | TIME | DISTANCE | PACE | HR |
|---------|------|----------|------|-----|
|  |  |  |  |  |
|  |  |  |  |  |
|  |  |  |  |  |
|  |  |  |  |  |

| SUPPLEMENTS & VITAMINS | SERVINGS | QUANTITY |
|------------------------|----------|----------|
|  |  |  |
|  |  |  |
|  |  |  |
|  |  |  |

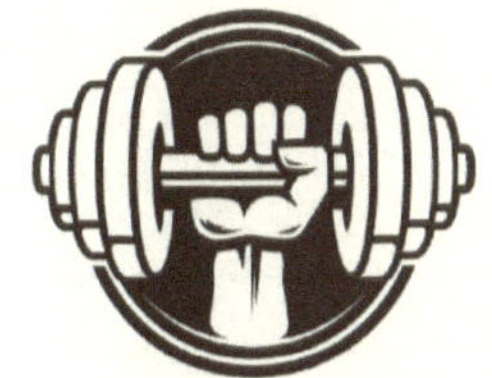

NAME:

DATE:

TIME START:

TIME END:

| WARM-UP | TIME | NOTES |
|---|---|---|
|  |  |  |
|  |  |  |
|  |  |  |

| EXERCISE: | SET 1 | | SET 2 | | SET 3 | | SET 4 | |
|---|---|---|---|---|---|---|---|---|
|  | REPS | WEIGHT | REPS | WEIGHT | REPS | WEIGHT | REPS | WEIGHT |
|  |  |  |  |  |  |  |  |  |
|  |  |  |  |  |  |  |  |  |
|  |  |  |  |  |  |  |  |  |
|  |  |  |  |  |  |  |  |  |
|  |  |  |  |  |  |  |  |  |
|  |  |  |  |  |  |  |  |  |
|  |  |  |  |  |  |  |  |  |
|  |  |  |  |  |  |  |  |  |
|  |  |  |  |  |  |  |  |  |
|  |  |  |  |  |  |  |  |  |
|  |  |  |  |  |  |  |  |  |

| CARDIO: | TIME | DISTANCE | PACE | HR |
|---|---|---|---|---|
|  |  |  |  |  |
|  |  |  |  |  |
|  |  |  |  |  |

| SUPPLEMENTS & VITAMINS | SERVINGS | QUANTITY |
|---|---|---|
|  |  |  |
|  |  |  |
|  |  |  |
|  |  |  |

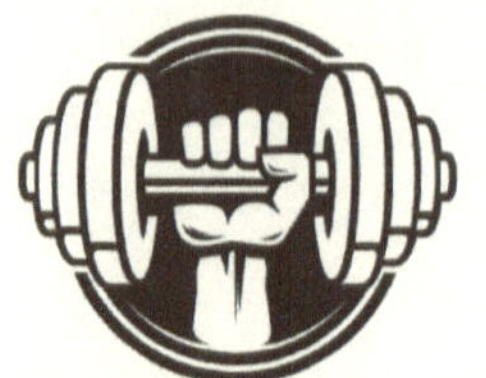

NAME:

DATE:

TIME START:

TIME END:

| WARM-UP | TIME | NOTES |
|---|---|---|
|  |  |  |
|  |  |  |
|  |  |  |
|  |  |  |

| EXERCISE: | SET 1 | | SET 2 | | SET 3 | | SET 4 | |
|---|---|---|---|---|---|---|---|---|
|  | REPS | WEIGHT | REPS | WEIGHT | REPS | WEIGHT | REPS | WEIGHT |
|  |  |  |  |  |  |  |  |  |
|  |  |  |  |  |  |  |  |  |
|  |  |  |  |  |  |  |  |  |
|  |  |  |  |  |  |  |  |  |
|  |  |  |  |  |  |  |  |  |
|  |  |  |  |  |  |  |  |  |
|  |  |  |  |  |  |  |  |  |
|  |  |  |  |  |  |  |  |  |
|  |  |  |  |  |  |  |  |  |
|  |  |  |  |  |  |  |  |  |
|  |  |  |  |  |  |  |  |  |
|  |  |  |  |  |  |  |  |  |

| CARDIO: | TIME | DISTANCE | PACE | HR |
|---|---|---|---|---|
|  |  |  |  |  |
|  |  |  |  |  |
|  |  |  |  |  |
|  |  |  |  |  |

| SUPPLEMENTS & VITAMINS | SERVINGS | QUANTITY |
|---|---|---|
|  |  |  |
|  |  |  |
|  |  |  |
|  |  |  |
|  |  |  |

NAME:

DATE:

TIME START:

TIME END:

| WARM-UP | TIME | NOTES |
|---------|------|-------|
|  |  |  |
|  |  |  |
|  |  |  |
|  |  |  |

| EXERCISE: | SET 1 | | SET 2 | | SET 3 | | SET 4 | |
|-----------|-------|--------|-------|--------|-------|--------|-------|--------|
|  | REPS | WEIGHT | REPS | WEIGHT | REPS | WEIGHT | REPS | WEIGHT |
|  |  |  |  |  |  |  |  |  |
|  |  |  |  |  |  |  |  |  |
|  |  |  |  |  |  |  |  |  |
|  |  |  |  |  |  |  |  |  |
|  |  |  |  |  |  |  |  |  |
|  |  |  |  |  |  |  |  |  |
|  |  |  |  |  |  |  |  |  |
|  |  |  |  |  |  |  |  |  |
|  |  |  |  |  |  |  |  |  |
|  |  |  |  |  |  |  |  |  |
|  |  |  |  |  |  |  |  |  |

| CARDIO: | TIME | DISTANCE | PACE | HR |
|---------|------|----------|------|-----|
|  |  |  |  |  |
|  |  |  |  |  |
|  |  |  |  |  |
|  |  |  |  |  |

| SUPPLEMENTS & VITAMINS | SERVINGS | QUANTITY |
|------------------------|----------|----------|
|  |  |  |
|  |  |  |
|  |  |  |
|  |  |  |
|  |  |  |

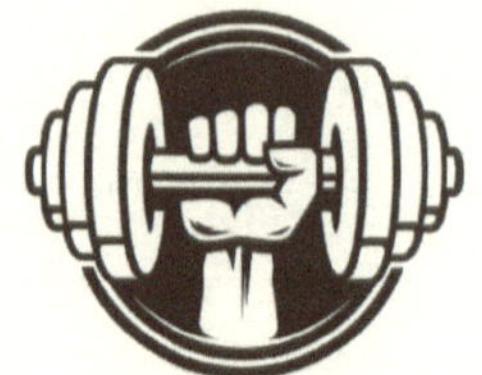

NAME:_______________________

DATE:_______________________

TIME START:_______________________

TIME END:_______________________

| WARM-UP | TIME | NOTES |
|---|---|---|
|  |  |  |
|  |  |  |
|  |  |  |
|  |  |  |

| EXERCISE: | SET 1 | | SET 2 | | SET 3 | | SET 4 | |
|---|---|---|---|---|---|---|---|---|
|  | REPS | WEIGHT | REPS | WEIGHT | REPS | WEIGHT | REPS | WEIGHT |
|  |  |  |  |  |  |  |  |  |
|  |  |  |  |  |  |  |  |  |
|  |  |  |  |  |  |  |  |  |
|  |  |  |  |  |  |  |  |  |
|  |  |  |  |  |  |  |  |  |
|  |  |  |  |  |  |  |  |  |
|  |  |  |  |  |  |  |  |  |
|  |  |  |  |  |  |  |  |  |
|  |  |  |  |  |  |  |  |  |
|  |  |  |  |  |  |  |  |  |
|  |  |  |  |  |  |  |  |  |

| CARDIO: | TIME | DISTANCE | PACE | HR |
|---|---|---|---|---|
|  |  |  |  |  |
|  |  |  |  |  |
|  |  |  |  |  |
|  |  |  |  |  |

| SUPPLEMENTS & VITAMINS | SERVINGS | QUANTITY |
|---|---|---|
|  |  |  |
|  |  |  |
|  |  |  |
|  |  |  |
|  |  |  |

NAME:_______________________

DATE:_______________________

TIME START:_______________________

TIME END:_______________________

| WARM-UP | TIME | NOTES |
|---|---|---|
|  |  |  |
|  |  |  |
|  |  |  |
|  |  |  |

| EXERCISE: | SET 1 | | SET 2 | | SET 3 | | SET 4 | |
|---|---|---|---|---|---|---|---|---|
|  | REPS | WEIGHT | REPS | WEIGHT | REPS | WEIGHT | REPS | WEIGHT |
|  |  |  |  |  |  |  |  |  |
|  |  |  |  |  |  |  |  |  |
|  |  |  |  |  |  |  |  |  |
|  |  |  |  |  |  |  |  |  |
|  |  |  |  |  |  |  |  |  |
|  |  |  |  |  |  |  |  |  |
|  |  |  |  |  |  |  |  |  |
|  |  |  |  |  |  |  |  |  |
|  |  |  |  |  |  |  |  |  |
|  |  |  |  |  |  |  |  |  |
|  |  |  |  |  |  |  |  |  |

| CARDIO: | TIME | DISTANCE | PACE | HR |
|---|---|---|---|---|
|  |  |  |  |  |
|  |  |  |  |  |
|  |  |  |  |  |
|  |  |  |  |  |

| SUPPLEMENTS & VITAMINS | SERVINGS | QUANTITY |
|---|---|---|
|  |  |  |
|  |  |  |
|  |  |  |
|  |  |  |
|  |  |  |

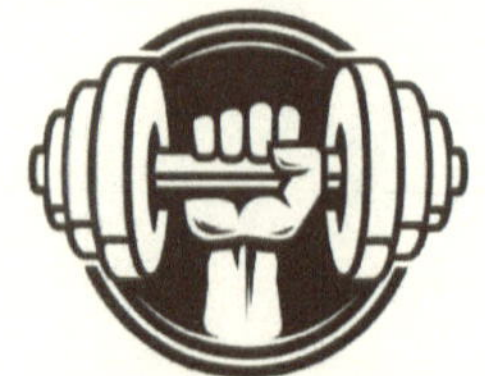

NAME:

DATE:

TIME START:

TIME END:

| WARM-UP | TIME | NOTES |
|---|---|---|
|  |  |  |
|  |  |  |
|  |  |  |
|  |  |  |

| EXERCISE: | SET 1 | | SET 2 | | SET 3 | | SET 4 | |
|---|---|---|---|---|---|---|---|---|
|  | REPS | WEIGHT | REPS | WEIGHT | REPS | WEIGHT | REPS | WEIGHT |
|  |  |  |  |  |  |  |  |  |
|  |  |  |  |  |  |  |  |  |
|  |  |  |  |  |  |  |  |  |
|  |  |  |  |  |  |  |  |  |
|  |  |  |  |  |  |  |  |  |
|  |  |  |  |  |  |  |  |  |
|  |  |  |  |  |  |  |  |  |
|  |  |  |  |  |  |  |  |  |
|  |  |  |  |  |  |  |  |  |
|  |  |  |  |  |  |  |  |  |
|  |  |  |  |  |  |  |  |  |

| CARDIO: | TIME | DISTANCE | PACE | HR |
|---|---|---|---|---|
|  |  |  |  |  |
|  |  |  |  |  |
|  |  |  |  |  |
|  |  |  |  |  |

| SUPPLEMENTS & VITAMINS | SERVINGS | QUANTITY |
|---|---|---|
|  |  |  |
|  |  |  |
|  |  |  |
|  |  |  |
|  |  |  |

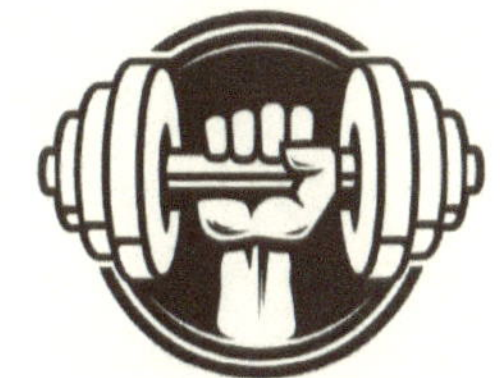



| WARM-UP | TIME | NOTES |
|---|---|---|
|  |  |  |
|  |  |  |
|  |  |  |
|  |  |  |

| EXERCISE: | SET 1 | | SET 2 | | SET 3 | | SET 4 | |
|---|---|---|---|---|---|---|---|---|
|  | REPS | WEIGHT | REPS | WEIGHT | REPS | WEIGHT | REPS | WEIGHT |
|  |  |  |  |  |  |  |  |  |
|  |  |  |  |  |  |  |  |  |
|  |  |  |  |  |  |  |  |  |
|  |  |  |  |  |  |  |  |  |
|  |  |  |  |  |  |  |  |  |
|  |  |  |  |  |  |  |  |  |
|  |  |  |  |  |  |  |  |  |
|  |  |  |  |  |  |  |  |  |
|  |  |  |  |  |  |  |  |  |
|  |  |  |  |  |  |  |  |  |
|  |  |  |  |  |  |  |  |  |
|  |  |  |  |  |  |  |  |  |

| CARDIO: | TIME | DISTANCE | PACE | HR |
|---|---|---|---|---|
|  |  |  |  |  |
|  |  |  |  |  |
|  |  |  |  |  |
|  |  |  |  |  |

| SUPPLEMENTS & VITAMINS | SERVINGS | QUANTITY |
|---|---|---|
|  |  |  |
|  |  |  |
|  |  |  |
|  |  |  |

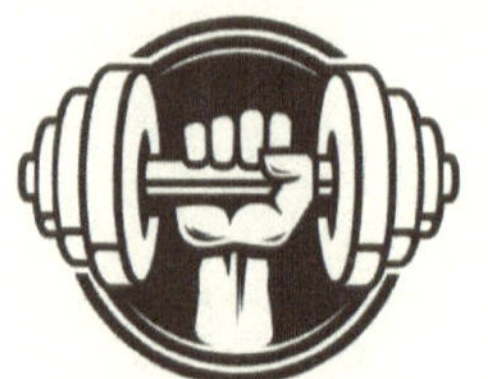

NAME:_______________________________

DATE:_______________________________

TIME START:_______________________________

TIME END:_______________________________

| WARM-UP | TIME | NOTES |
|---|---|---|
|  |  |  |
|  |  |  |
|  |  |  |
|  |  |  |

| EXERCISE: | SET 1 | | SET 2 | | SET 3 | | SET 4 | |
|---|---|---|---|---|---|---|---|---|
|  | REPS | WEIGHT | REPS | WEIGHT | REPS | WEIGHT | REPS | WEIGHT |
|  |  |  |  |  |  |  |  |  |
|  |  |  |  |  |  |  |  |  |
|  |  |  |  |  |  |  |  |  |
|  |  |  |  |  |  |  |  |  |
|  |  |  |  |  |  |  |  |  |
|  |  |  |  |  |  |  |  |  |
|  |  |  |  |  |  |  |  |  |
|  |  |  |  |  |  |  |  |  |
|  |  |  |  |  |  |  |  |  |
|  |  |  |  |  |  |  |  |  |
|  |  |  |  |  |  |  |  |  |

| CARDIO: | TIME | DISTANCE | PACE | HR |
|---|---|---|---|---|
|  |  |  |  |  |
|  |  |  |  |  |
|  |  |  |  |  |
|  |  |  |  |  |

| SUPPLEMENTS & VITAMINS | SERVINGS | QUANTITY |
|---|---|---|
|  |  |  |
|  |  |  |
|  |  |  |
|  |  |  |

NAME:______________________________

DATE:______________________________

TIME START:______________________________

TIME END:______________________________

| WARM-UP | TIME | NOTES |
|---|---|---|
|  |  |  |
|  |  |  |
|  |  |  |
|  |  |  |

| EXERCISE: | SET 1 | | SET 2 | | SET 3 | | SET 4 | |
|---|---|---|---|---|---|---|---|---|
| | REPS | WEIGHT | REPS | WEIGHT | REPS | WEIGHT | REPS | WEIGHT |
|  |  |  |  |  |  |  |  |  |
|  |  |  |  |  |  |  |  |  |
|  |  |  |  |  |  |  |  |  |
|  |  |  |  |  |  |  |  |  |
|  |  |  |  |  |  |  |  |  |
|  |  |  |  |  |  |  |  |  |
|  |  |  |  |  |  |  |  |  |
|  |  |  |  |  |  |  |  |  |
|  |  |  |  |  |  |  |  |  |
|  |  |  |  |  |  |  |  |  |
|  |  |  |  |  |  |  |  |  |
|  |  |  |  |  |  |  |  |  |

| CARDIO: | TIME | DISTANCE | PACE | HR |
|---|---|---|---|---|
|  |  |  |  |  |
|  |  |  |  |  |
|  |  |  |  |  |
|  |  |  |  |  |

| SUPPLEMENTS & VITAMINS | SERVINGS | QUANTITY |
|---|---|---|
|  |  |  |
|  |  |  |
|  |  |  |
|  |  |  |
|  |  |  |

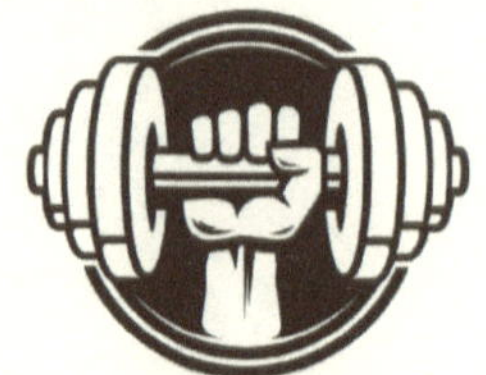

**NAME:**_______________________________

**DATE:**_______________________________

**TIME START:**_______________________________

**TIME END:**_______________________________

| WARM-UP | TIME | NOTES |
|---|---|---|
|  |  |  |
|  |  |  |
|  |  |  |
|  |  |  |

| EXERCISE: | SET 1 | | SET 2 | | SET 3 | | SET 4 | |
|---|---|---|---|---|---|---|---|---|
|  | REPS | WEIGHT | REPS | WEIGHT | REPS | WEIGHT | REPS | WEIGHT |
|  |  |  |  |  |  |  |  |  |
|  |  |  |  |  |  |  |  |  |
|  |  |  |  |  |  |  |  |  |
|  |  |  |  |  |  |  |  |  |
|  |  |  |  |  |  |  |  |  |
|  |  |  |  |  |  |  |  |  |
|  |  |  |  |  |  |  |  |  |
|  |  |  |  |  |  |  |  |  |
|  |  |  |  |  |  |  |  |  |
|  |  |  |  |  |  |  |  |  |
|  |  |  |  |  |  |  |  |  |

| CARDIO: | TIME | DISTANCE | PACE | HR |
|---|---|---|---|---|
|  |  |  |  |  |
|  |  |  |  |  |
|  |  |  |  |  |
|  |  |  |  |  |

| SUPPLEMENTS & VITAMINS | SERVINGS | QUANTITY |
|---|---|---|
|  |  |  |
|  |  |  |
|  |  |  |
|  |  |  |
|  |  |  |

| NAME: | |
| --- | --- |
| DATE: | |
| TIME START: | |
| TIME END: | |

| WARM-UP | TIME | NOTES |
| --- | --- | --- |
| | | |
| | | |
| | | |
| | | |

| EXERCISE: | SET 1 | | SET 2 | | SET 3 | | SET 4 | |
| --- | --- | --- | --- | --- | --- | --- | --- | --- |
| | REPS | WEIGHT | REPS | WEIGHT | REPS | WEIGHT | REPS | WEIGHT |
| | | | | | | | | |
| | | | | | | | | |
| | | | | | | | | |
| | | | | | | | | |
| | | | | | | | | |
| | | | | | | | | |
| | | | | | | | | |
| | | | | | | | | |
| | | | | | | | | |
| | | | | | | | | |
| | | | | | | | | |
| | | | | | | | | |
| | | | | | | | | |

| CARDIO: | TIME | DISTANCE | PACE | HR |
| --- | --- | --- | --- | --- |
| | | | | |
| | | | | |
| | | | | |
| | | | | |

| SUPPLEMENTS & VITAMINS | SERVINGS | QUANTITY |
| --- | --- | --- |
| | | |
| | | |
| | | |
| | | |
| | | |

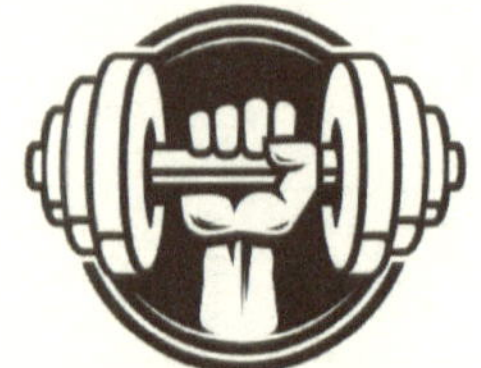

NAME:

DATE:

TIME START:

TIME END:

| WARM-UP | TIME | NOTES |
|---|---|---|
|  |  |  |
|  |  |  |
|  |  |  |
|  |  |  |

| EXERCISE: | SET 1 | | SET 2 | | SET 3 | | SET 4 | |
|---|---|---|---|---|---|---|---|---|
|  | REPS | WEIGHT | REPS | WEIGHT | REPS | WEIGHT | REPS | WEIGHT |
|  |  |  |  |  |  |  |  |  |
|  |  |  |  |  |  |  |  |  |
|  |  |  |  |  |  |  |  |  |
|  |  |  |  |  |  |  |  |  |
|  |  |  |  |  |  |  |  |  |
|  |  |  |  |  |  |  |  |  |
|  |  |  |  |  |  |  |  |  |
|  |  |  |  |  |  |  |  |  |
|  |  |  |  |  |  |  |  |  |
|  |  |  |  |  |  |  |  |  |
|  |  |  |  |  |  |  |  |  |

| CARDIO: | TIME | DISTANCE | PACE | HR |
|---|---|---|---|---|
|  |  |  |  |  |
|  |  |  |  |  |
|  |  |  |  |  |
|  |  |  |  |  |

| SUPPLEMENTS & VITAMINS | SERVINGS | QUANTITY |
|---|---|---|
|  |  |  |
|  |  |  |
|  |  |  |
|  |  |  |
|  |  |  |

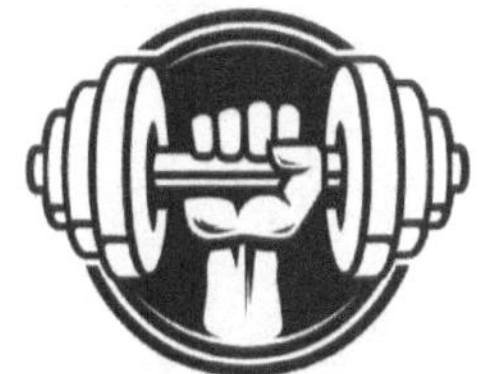

NAME:___________________________

DATE:___________________________

TIME START:___________________________

TIME END:___________________________

| WARM-UP | TIME | NOTES |
|---------|------|-------|
|  |  |  |
|  |  |  |
|  |  |  |
|  |  |  |

| EXERCISE: | SET 1 | | SET 2 | | SET 3 | | SET 4 | |
|-----------|-------|--------|-------|--------|-------|--------|-------|--------|
|  | REPS | WEIGHT | REPS | WEIGHT | REPS | WEIGHT | REPS | WEIGHT |
|  |  |  |  |  |  |  |  |  |
|  |  |  |  |  |  |  |  |  |
|  |  |  |  |  |  |  |  |  |
|  |  |  |  |  |  |  |  |  |
|  |  |  |  |  |  |  |  |  |
|  |  |  |  |  |  |  |  |  |
|  |  |  |  |  |  |  |  |  |
|  |  |  |  |  |  |  |  |  |
|  |  |  |  |  |  |  |  |  |
|  |  |  |  |  |  |  |  |  |
|  |  |  |  |  |  |  |  |  |
|  |  |  |  |  |  |  |  |  |

| CARDIO: | TIME | DISTANCE | PACE | HR |
|---------|------|----------|------|----|
|  |  |  |  |  |
|  |  |  |  |  |
|  |  |  |  |  |
|  |  |  |  |  |

| SUPPLEMENTS & VITAMINS | SERVINGS | QUANTITY |
|------------------------|----------|----------|
|  |  |  |
|  |  |  |
|  |  |  |
|  |  |  |
|  |  |  |

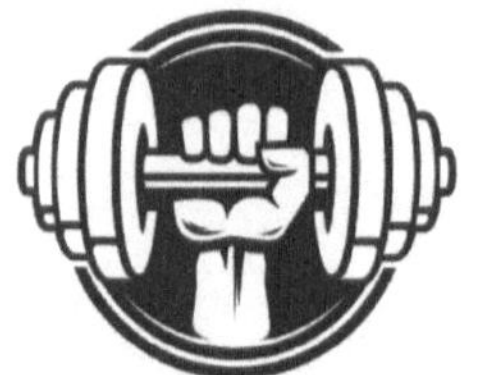

NAME:_______________________

DATE:_______________________

TIME START:_________________

TIME END:___________________

| WARM-UP | TIME | NOTES |
|---|---|---|
|  |  |  |
|  |  |  |
|  |  |  |
|  |  |  |

| EXERCISE: | SET 1 | | SET 2 | | SET 3 | | SET 4 | |
|---|---|---|---|---|---|---|---|---|
|  | REPS | WEIGHT | REPS | WEIGHT | REPS | WEIGHT | REPS | WEIGHT |
|  |  |  |  |  |  |  |  |  |
|  |  |  |  |  |  |  |  |  |
|  |  |  |  |  |  |  |  |  |
|  |  |  |  |  |  |  |  |  |
|  |  |  |  |  |  |  |  |  |
|  |  |  |  |  |  |  |  |  |
|  |  |  |  |  |  |  |  |  |
|  |  |  |  |  |  |  |  |  |
|  |  |  |  |  |  |  |  |  |
|  |  |  |  |  |  |  |  |  |

| CARDIO: | TIME | DISTANCE | PACE | HR |
|---|---|---|---|---|
|  |  |  |  |  |
|  |  |  |  |  |
|  |  |  |  |  |
|  |  |  |  |  |

| SUPPLEMENTS & VITAMINS | SERVINGS | QUANTITY |
|---|---|---|
|  |  |  |
|  |  |  |
|  |  |  |
|  |  |  |
|  |  |  |

NAME:_______________________

DATE:_______________________

TIME START:_______________________

TIME END:_______________________

| WARM-UP | TIME | NOTES |
|---|---|---|
| | | |
| | | |
| | | |
| | | |

| EXERCISE: | SET 1 | | SET 2 | | SET 3 | | SET 4 | |
|---|---|---|---|---|---|---|---|---|
| | REPS | WEIGHT | REPS | WEIGHT | REPS | WEIGHT | REPS | WEIGHT |
| | | | | | | | | |
| | | | | | | | | |
| | | | | | | | | |
| | | | | | | | | |
| | | | | | | | | |
| | | | | | | | | |
| | | | | | | | | |
| | | | | | | | | |
| | | | | | | | | |
| | | | | | | | | |
| | | | | | | | | |

| CARDIO: | TIME | DISTANCE | PACE | HR |
|---|---|---|---|---|
| | | | | |
| | | | | |
| | | | | |
| | | | | |

| SUPPLEMENTS & VITAMINS | SERVINGS | QUANTITY |
|---|---|---|
| | | |
| | | |
| | | |
| | | |
| | | |

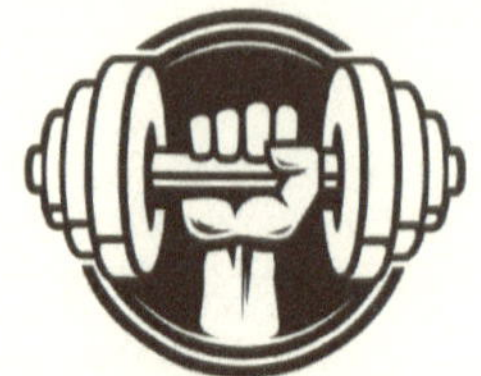

NAME:________________________________

DATE:________________________________

TIME START:__________________________

TIME END:____________________________

| WARM-UP | TIME | NOTES |
|---|---|---|
|  |  |  |
|  |  |  |
|  |  |  |
|  |  |  |

| EXERCISE: | SET 1 | | SET 2 | | SET 3 | | SET 4 | |
|---|---|---|---|---|---|---|---|---|
|  | REPS | WEIGHT | REPS | WEIGHT | REPS | WEIGHT | REPS | WEIGHT |
|  |  |  |  |  |  |  |  |  |
|  |  |  |  |  |  |  |  |  |
|  |  |  |  |  |  |  |  |  |
|  |  |  |  |  |  |  |  |  |
|  |  |  |  |  |  |  |  |  |
|  |  |  |  |  |  |  |  |  |
|  |  |  |  |  |  |  |  |  |
|  |  |  |  |  |  |  |  |  |
|  |  |  |  |  |  |  |  |  |
|  |  |  |  |  |  |  |  |  |
|  |  |  |  |  |  |  |  |  |
|  |  |  |  |  |  |  |  |  |

| CARDIO: | TIME | DISTANCE | PACE | HR |
|---|---|---|---|---|
|  |  |  |  |  |
|  |  |  |  |  |
|  |  |  |  |  |
|  |  |  |  |  |

| SUPPLEMENTS & VITAMINS | SERVINGS | QUANTITY |
|---|---|---|
|  |  |  |
|  |  |  |
|  |  |  |
|  |  |  |

NAME:_________________________________

DATE:_________________________________

TIME START:_________________________________

TIME END:_________________________________

| WARM-UP | TIME | NOTES |
|---------|------|-------|
|  |  |  |
|  |  |  |
|  |  |  |
|  |  |  |

| EXERCISE: | SET 1 | | SET 2 | | SET 3 | | SET 4 | |
|-----------|-------|--------|-------|--------|-------|--------|-------|--------|
|  | REPS | WEIGHT | REPS | WEIGHT | REPS | WEIGHT | REPS | WEIGHT |
|  |  |  |  |  |  |  |  |  |
|  |  |  |  |  |  |  |  |  |
|  |  |  |  |  |  |  |  |  |
|  |  |  |  |  |  |  |  |  |
|  |  |  |  |  |  |  |  |  |
|  |  |  |  |  |  |  |  |  |
|  |  |  |  |  |  |  |  |  |
|  |  |  |  |  |  |  |  |  |
|  |  |  |  |  |  |  |  |  |
|  |  |  |  |  |  |  |  |  |

| CARDIO: | TIME | DISTANCE | PACE | HR |
|---------|------|----------|------|----|
|  |  |  |  |  |
|  |  |  |  |  |
|  |  |  |  |  |
|  |  |  |  |  |

| SUPPLEMENTS & VITAMINS | SERVINGS | QUANTITY |
|------------------------|----------|----------|
|  |  |  |
|  |  |  |
|  |  |  |
|  |  |  |
|  |  |  |

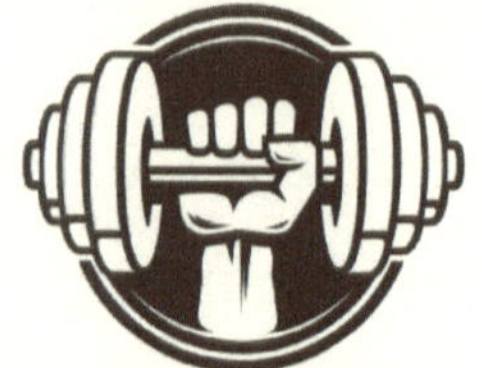

NAME:

DATE:

TIME START:

TIME END:

| WARM-UP | TIME | NOTES |
|---|---|---|
|  |  |  |
|  |  |  |
|  |  |  |
|  |  |  |

| EXERCISE: | SET 1 | | SET 2 | | SET 3 | | SET 4 | |
|---|---|---|---|---|---|---|---|---|
|  | REPS | WEIGHT | REPS | WEIGHT | REPS | WEIGHT | REPS | WEIGHT |
|  |  |  |  |  |  |  |  |  |
|  |  |  |  |  |  |  |  |  |
|  |  |  |  |  |  |  |  |  |
|  |  |  |  |  |  |  |  |  |
|  |  |  |  |  |  |  |  |  |
|  |  |  |  |  |  |  |  |  |
|  |  |  |  |  |  |  |  |  |
|  |  |  |  |  |  |  |  |  |
|  |  |  |  |  |  |  |  |  |
|  |  |  |  |  |  |  |  |  |
|  |  |  |  |  |  |  |  |  |
|  |  |  |  |  |  |  |  |  |

| CARDIO: | TIME | DISTANCE | PACE | HR |
|---|---|---|---|---|
|  |  |  |  |  |
|  |  |  |  |  |
|  |  |  |  |  |
|  |  |  |  |  |

| SUPPLEMENTS & VITAMINS | SERVINGS | QUANTITY |
|---|---|---|
|  |  |  |
|  |  |  |
|  |  |  |
|  |  |  |
|  |  |  |

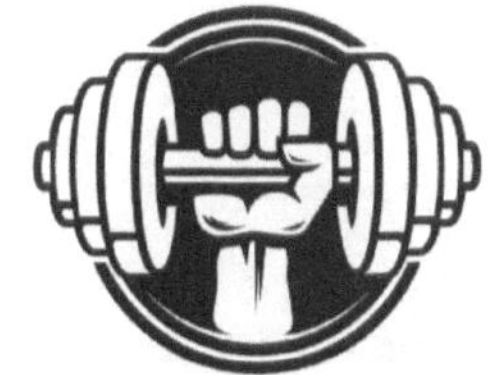

NAME:______________________________

DATE:______________________________

TIME START:______________________________

TIME END:______________________________

| WARM-UP | TIME | NOTES |
|---|---|---|
|  |  |  |
|  |  |  |
|  |  |  |
|  |  |  |

| EXERCISE: | SET 1 | | SET 2 | | SET 3 | | SET 4 | |
|---|---|---|---|---|---|---|---|---|
|  | REPS | WEIGHT | REPS | WEIGHT | REPS | WEIGHT | REPS | WEIGHT |
|  |  |  |  |  |  |  |  |  |
|  |  |  |  |  |  |  |  |  |
|  |  |  |  |  |  |  |  |  |
|  |  |  |  |  |  |  |  |  |
|  |  |  |  |  |  |  |  |  |
|  |  |  |  |  |  |  |  |  |
|  |  |  |  |  |  |  |  |  |
|  |  |  |  |  |  |  |  |  |
|  |  |  |  |  |  |  |  |  |
|  |  |  |  |  |  |  |  |  |
|  |  |  |  |  |  |  |  |  |
|  |  |  |  |  |  |  |  |  |

| CARDIO: | TIME | DISTANCE | PACE | HR |
|---|---|---|---|---|
|  |  |  |  |  |
|  |  |  |  |  |
|  |  |  |  |  |
|  |  |  |  |  |

| SUPPLEMENTS & VITAMINS | SERVINGS | QUANTITY |
|---|---|---|
|  |  |  |
|  |  |  |
|  |  |  |
|  |  |  |
|  |  |  |

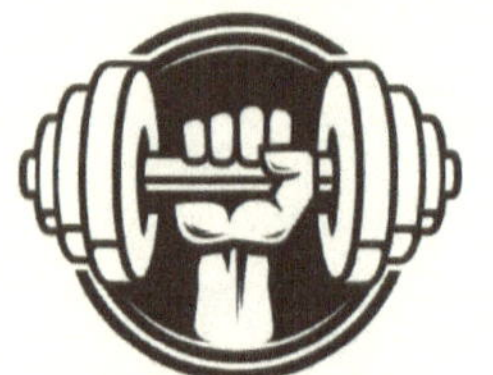

NAME:_______________________________

DATE:_______________________________

TIME START:_________________________

TIME END:___________________________

| WARM-UP | TIME | NOTES |
|---|---|---|
|  |  |  |
|  |  |  |
|  |  |  |
|  |  |  |

| EXERCISE: | SET 1 | | SET 2 | | SET 3 | | SET 4 | |
|---|---|---|---|---|---|---|---|---|
|  | REPS | WEIGHT | REPS | WEIGHT | REPS | WEIGHT | REPS | WEIGHT |
|  |  |  |  |  |  |  |  |  |
|  |  |  |  |  |  |  |  |  |
|  |  |  |  |  |  |  |  |  |
|  |  |  |  |  |  |  |  |  |
|  |  |  |  |  |  |  |  |  |
|  |  |  |  |  |  |  |  |  |
|  |  |  |  |  |  |  |  |  |
|  |  |  |  |  |  |  |  |  |
|  |  |  |  |  |  |  |  |  |
|  |  |  |  |  |  |  |  |  |
|  |  |  |  |  |  |  |  |  |

| CARDIO: | TIME | DISTANCE | PACE | HR |
|---|---|---|---|---|
|  |  |  |  |  |
|  |  |  |  |  |
|  |  |  |  |  |
|  |  |  |  |  |

| SUPPLEMENTS & VITAMINS | SERVINGS | QUANTITY |
|---|---|---|
|  |  |  |
|  |  |  |
|  |  |  |
|  |  |  |

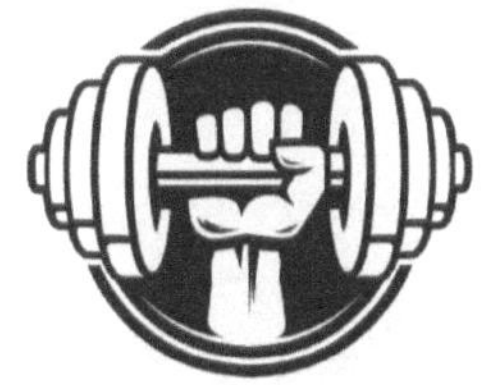

NAME:_______________________________

DATE:_______________________________

TIME START:_______________________________

TIME END:_______________________________

| WARM-UP | TIME | NOTES |
|---|---|---|
|  |  |  |
|  |  |  |
|  |  |  |
|  |  |  |

| EXERCISE: | SET 1 | | SET 2 | | SET 3 | | SET 4 | |
|---|---|---|---|---|---|---|---|---|
|  | REPS | WEIGHT | REPS | WEIGHT | REPS | WEIGHT | REPS | WEIGHT |
|  |  |  |  |  |  |  |  |  |
|  |  |  |  |  |  |  |  |  |
|  |  |  |  |  |  |  |  |  |
|  |  |  |  |  |  |  |  |  |
|  |  |  |  |  |  |  |  |  |
|  |  |  |  |  |  |  |  |  |
|  |  |  |  |  |  |  |  |  |
|  |  |  |  |  |  |  |  |  |
|  |  |  |  |  |  |  |  |  |
|  |  |  |  |  |  |  |  |  |
|  |  |  |  |  |  |  |  |  |
|  |  |  |  |  |  |  |  |  |

| CARDIO: | TIME | DISTANCE | PACE | HR |
|---|---|---|---|---|
|  |  |  |  |  |
|  |  |  |  |  |
|  |  |  |  |  |
|  |  |  |  |  |

| SUPPLEMENTS & VITAMINS | SERVINGS | QUANTITY |
|---|---|---|
|  |  |  |
|  |  |  |
|  |  |  |
|  |  |  |
|  |  |  |

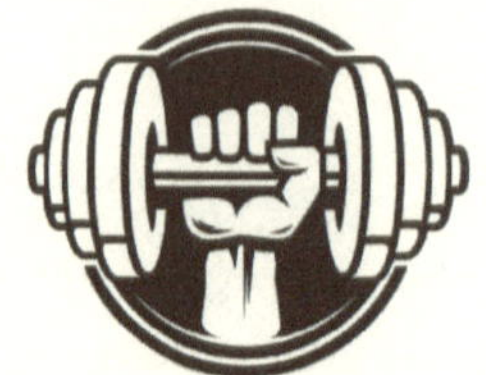

**NAME:**

**DATE:**

**TIME START:**

**TIME END:**

| WARM-UP | TIME | NOTES |
|---|---|---|
| | | |
| | | |
| | | |
| | | |

| EXERCISE: | SET 1 | | SET 2 | | SET 3 | | SET 4 | |
|---|---|---|---|---|---|---|---|---|
| | REPS | WEIGHT | REPS | WEIGHT | REPS | WEIGHT | REPS | WEIGHT |
| | | | | | | | | |
| | | | | | | | | |
| | | | | | | | | |
| | | | | | | | | |
| | | | | | | | | |
| | | | | | | | | |
| | | | | | | | | |
| | | | | | | | | |
| | | | | | | | | |
| | | | | | | | | |
| | | | | | | | | |
| | | | | | | | | |

| CARDIO: | TIME | DISTANCE | PACE | HR |
|---|---|---|---|---|
| | | | | |
| | | | | |
| | | | | |
| | | | | |

| SUPPLEMENTS & VITAMINS | SERVINGS | QUANTITY |
|---|---|---|
| | | |
| | | |
| | | |
| | | |
| | | |

NAME:

DATE:

TIME START:

TIME END:

| WARM-UP | TIME | NOTES |
|---|---|---|
|  |  |  |
|  |  |  |
|  |  |  |
|  |  |  |

| EXERCISE: | SET 1 | | SET 2 | | SET 3 | | SET 4 | |
|---|---|---|---|---|---|---|---|---|
|  | REPS | WEIGHT | REPS | WEIGHT | REPS | WEIGHT | REPS | WEIGHT |
|  |  |  |  |  |  |  |  |  |
|  |  |  |  |  |  |  |  |  |
|  |  |  |  |  |  |  |  |  |
|  |  |  |  |  |  |  |  |  |
|  |  |  |  |  |  |  |  |  |
|  |  |  |  |  |  |  |  |  |
|  |  |  |  |  |  |  |  |  |
|  |  |  |  |  |  |  |  |  |
|  |  |  |  |  |  |  |  |  |
|  |  |  |  |  |  |  |  |  |
|  |  |  |  |  |  |  |  |  |
|  |  |  |  |  |  |  |  |  |

| CARDIO: | TIME | DISTANCE | PACE | HR |
|---|---|---|---|---|
|  |  |  |  |  |
|  |  |  |  |  |
|  |  |  |  |  |
|  |  |  |  |  |

| SUPPLEMENTS & VITAMINS | SERVINGS | QUANTITY |
|---|---|---|
|  |  |  |
|  |  |  |
|  |  |  |
|  |  |  |

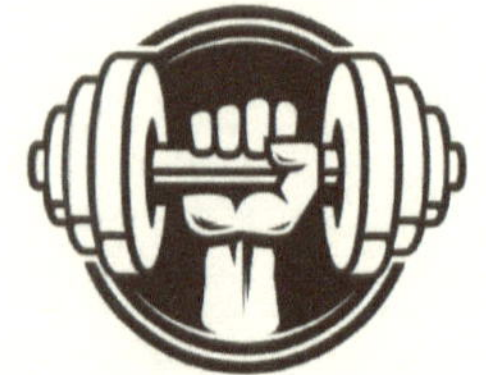

NAME:_______________________________

DATE:_______________________________

TIME START:_________________________

TIME END:___________________________

| WARM-UP | TIME | NOTES |
|---------|------|-------|
| | | |
| | | |
| | | |
| | | |

| EXERCISE: | SET 1 | | SET 2 | | SET 3 | | SET 4 | |
|-----------|-------|--------|-------|--------|-------|--------|-------|--------|
| | REPS | WEIGHT | REPS | WEIGHT | REPS | WEIGHT | REPS | WEIGHT |
| | | | | | | | | |
| | | | | | | | | |
| | | | | | | | | |
| | | | | | | | | |
| | | | | | | | | |
| | | | | | | | | |
| | | | | | | | | |
| | | | | | | | | |
| | | | | | | | | |
| | | | | | | | | |
| | | | | | | | | |

| CARDIO: | TIME | DISTANCE | PACE | HR |
|---------|------|----------|------|----|
| | | | | |
| | | | | |
| | | | | |
| | | | | |

| SUPPLEMENTS & VITAMINS | SERVINGS | QUANTITY |
|------------------------|----------|----------|
| | | |
| | | |
| | | |
| | | |

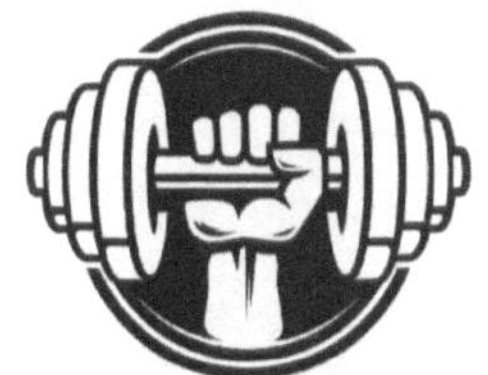

**NAME:**_______________________________

**DATE:**_______________________________

**TIME START:**_______________________________

**TIME END:**_______________________________

| WARM-UP | TIME | NOTES |
|---|---|---|
| | | |
| | | |
| | | |
| | | |

| EXERCISE: | SET 1 | | SET 2 | | SET 3 | | SET 4 | |
|---|---|---|---|---|---|---|---|---|
| | REPS | WEIGHT | REPS | WEIGHT | REPS | WEIGHT | REPS | WEIGHT |
| | | | | | | | | |
| | | | | | | | | |
| | | | | | | | | |
| | | | | | | | | |
| | | | | | | | | |
| | | | | | | | | |
| | | | | | | | | |
| | | | | | | | | |
| | | | | | | | | |
| | | | | | | | | |
| | | | | | | | | |
| | | | | | | | | |

| CARDIO: | TIME | DISTANCE | PACE | HR |
|---|---|---|---|---|
| | | | | |
| | | | | |
| | | | | |
| | | | | |

| SUPPLEMENTS & VITAMINS | SERVINGS | QUANTITY |
|---|---|---|
| | | |
| | | |
| | | |
| | | |
| | | |

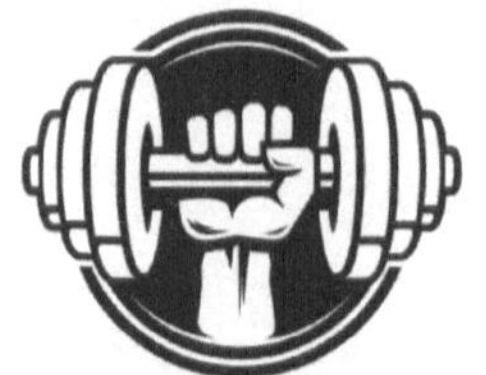

NAME:

DATE:

TIME START:

TIME END:

| WARM-UP | TIME | NOTES |
|---|---|---|
|  |  |  |
|  |  |  |
|  |  |  |

| EXERCISE: | SET 1 | | SET 2 | | SET 3 | | SET 4 | |
|---|---|---|---|---|---|---|---|---|
|  | REPS | WEIGHT | REPS | WEIGHT | REPS | WEIGHT | REPS | WEIGHT |
|  |  |  |  |  |  |  |  |  |
|  |  |  |  |  |  |  |  |  |
|  |  |  |  |  |  |  |  |  |
|  |  |  |  |  |  |  |  |  |
|  |  |  |  |  |  |  |  |  |
|  |  |  |  |  |  |  |  |  |
|  |  |  |  |  |  |  |  |  |
|  |  |  |  |  |  |  |  |  |
|  |  |  |  |  |  |  |  |  |
|  |  |  |  |  |  |  |  |  |

| CARDIO: | TIME | DISTANCE | PACE | HR |
|---|---|---|---|---|
|  |  |  |  |  |
|  |  |  |  |  |
|  |  |  |  |  |
|  |  |  |  |  |

| SUPPLEMENTS & VITAMINS | SERVINGS | QUANTITY |
|---|---|---|
|  |  |  |
|  |  |  |
|  |  |  |
|  |  |  |

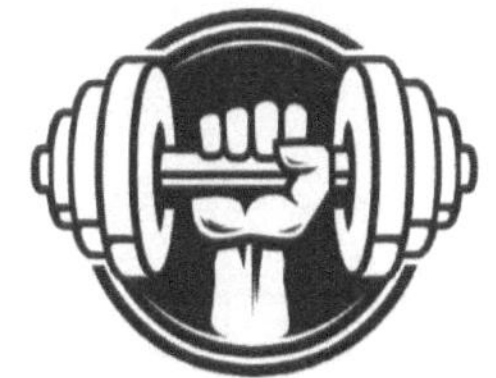

NAME:

DATE:

TIME START:

TIME END:

| WARM-UP | TIME | NOTES |
|---|---|---|
|  |  |  |
|  |  |  |
|  |  |  |
|  |  |  |

| EXERCISE: | SET 1 | | SET 2 | | SET 3 | | SET 4 | |
|---|---|---|---|---|---|---|---|---|
|  | REPS | WEIGHT | REPS | WEIGHT | REPS | WEIGHT | REPS | WEIGHT |
|  |  |  |  |  |  |  |  |  |
|  |  |  |  |  |  |  |  |  |
|  |  |  |  |  |  |  |  |  |
|  |  |  |  |  |  |  |  |  |
|  |  |  |  |  |  |  |  |  |
|  |  |  |  |  |  |  |  |  |
|  |  |  |  |  |  |  |  |  |
|  |  |  |  |  |  |  |  |  |
|  |  |  |  |  |  |  |  |  |
|  |  |  |  |  |  |  |  |  |
|  |  |  |  |  |  |  |  |  |
|  |  |  |  |  |  |  |  |  |

| CARDIO: | TIME | DISTANCE | PACE | HR |
|---|---|---|---|---|
|  |  |  |  |  |
|  |  |  |  |  |
|  |  |  |  |  |
|  |  |  |  |  |

| SUPPLEMENTS & VITAMINS | SERVINGS | QUANTITY |
|---|---|---|
|  |  |  |
|  |  |  |
|  |  |  |
|  |  |  |
|  |  |  |

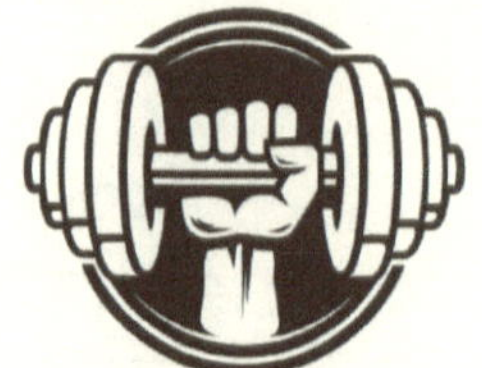

NAME:_______________________________

DATE:_______________________________

TIME START:_________________________

TIME END:___________________________

| WARM-UP | TIME | NOTES |
|---|---|---|
|  |  |  |
|  |  |  |
|  |  |  |
|  |  |  |

| EXERCISE: | SET 1 | | SET 2 | | SET 3 | | SET 4 | |
|---|---|---|---|---|---|---|---|---|
|  | REPS | WEIGHT | REPS | WEIGHT | REPS | WEIGHT | REPS | WEIGHT |
|  |  |  |  |  |  |  |  |  |
|  |  |  |  |  |  |  |  |  |
|  |  |  |  |  |  |  |  |  |
|  |  |  |  |  |  |  |  |  |
|  |  |  |  |  |  |  |  |  |
|  |  |  |  |  |  |  |  |  |
|  |  |  |  |  |  |  |  |  |
|  |  |  |  |  |  |  |  |  |
|  |  |  |  |  |  |  |  |  |
|  |  |  |  |  |  |  |  |  |
|  |  |  |  |  |  |  |  |  |
|  |  |  |  |  |  |  |  |  |

| CARDIO: | TIME | DISTANCE | PACE | HR |
|---|---|---|---|---|
|  |  |  |  |  |
|  |  |  |  |  |
|  |  |  |  |  |
|  |  |  |  |  |

| SUPPLEMENTS & VITAMINS | SERVINGS | QUANTITY |
|---|---|---|
|  |  |  |
|  |  |  |
|  |  |  |
|  |  |  |

NAME:

DATE:

TIME START:

TIME END:

| WARM-UP | TIME | NOTES |
|---|---|---|
|  |  |  |
|  |  |  |
|  |  |  |
|  |  |  |

| EXERCISE: | SET 1 | | SET 2 | | SET 3 | | SET 4 | |
|---|---|---|---|---|---|---|---|---|
|  | REPS | WEIGHT | REPS | WEIGHT | REPS | WEIGHT | REPS | WEIGHT |
|  |  |  |  |  |  |  |  |  |
|  |  |  |  |  |  |  |  |  |
|  |  |  |  |  |  |  |  |  |
|  |  |  |  |  |  |  |  |  |
|  |  |  |  |  |  |  |  |  |
|  |  |  |  |  |  |  |  |  |
|  |  |  |  |  |  |  |  |  |
|  |  |  |  |  |  |  |  |  |
|  |  |  |  |  |  |  |  |  |
|  |  |  |  |  |  |  |  |  |
|  |  |  |  |  |  |  |  |  |

| CARDIO: | TIME | DISTANCE | PACE | HR |
|---|---|---|---|---|
|  |  |  |  |  |
|  |  |  |  |  |
|  |  |  |  |  |
|  |  |  |  |  |

| SUPPLEMENTS & VITAMINS | SERVINGS | QUANTITY |
|---|---|---|
|  |  |  |
|  |  |  |
|  |  |  |
|  |  |  |
|  |  |  |

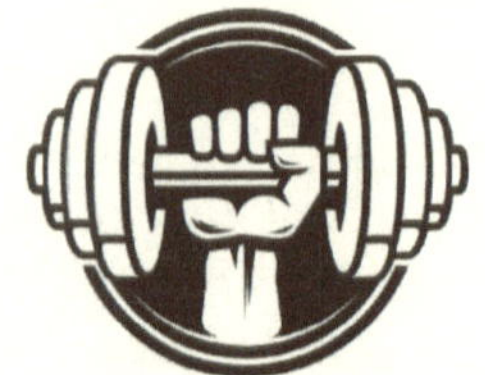

NAME:

DATE:

TIME START:

TIME END:

| WARM-UP | TIME | NOTES |
|---|---|---|
|  |  |  |
|  |  |  |
|  |  |  |
|  |  |  |

| EXERCISE: | SET 1 | | SET 2 | | SET 3 | | SET 4 | |
|---|---|---|---|---|---|---|---|---|
|  | REPS | WEIGHT | REPS | WEIGHT | REPS | WEIGHT | REPS | WEIGHT |
|  |  |  |  |  |  |  |  |  |
|  |  |  |  |  |  |  |  |  |
|  |  |  |  |  |  |  |  |  |
|  |  |  |  |  |  |  |  |  |
|  |  |  |  |  |  |  |  |  |
|  |  |  |  |  |  |  |  |  |
|  |  |  |  |  |  |  |  |  |
|  |  |  |  |  |  |  |  |  |
|  |  |  |  |  |  |  |  |  |
|  |  |  |  |  |  |  |  |  |
|  |  |  |  |  |  |  |  |  |
|  |  |  |  |  |  |  |  |  |

| CARDIO: | TIME | DISTANCE | PACE | HR |
|---|---|---|---|---|
|  |  |  |  |  |
|  |  |  |  |  |
|  |  |  |  |  |
|  |  |  |  |  |

| SUPPLEMENTS & VITAMINS | SERVINGS | QUANTITY |
|---|---|---|
|  |  |  |
|  |  |  |
|  |  |  |
|  |  |  |
|  |  |  |

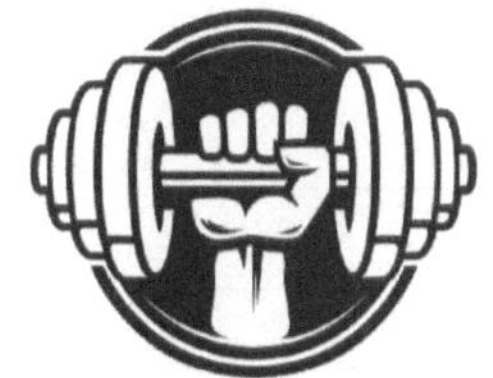

**NAME:**_______________________

**DATE:**_______________________

**TIME START:**_______________________

**TIME END:**_______________________

| WARM-UP | TIME | NOTES |
|---|---|---|
|  |  |  |
|  |  |  |
|  |  |  |
|  |  |  |

| EXERCISE: | SET 1 | | SET 2 | | SET 3 | | SET 4 | |
|---|---|---|---|---|---|---|---|---|
|  | REPS | WEIGHT | REPS | WEIGHT | REPS | WEIGHT | REPS | WEIGHT |
|  |  |  |  |  |  |  |  |  |
|  |  |  |  |  |  |  |  |  |
|  |  |  |  |  |  |  |  |  |
|  |  |  |  |  |  |  |  |  |
|  |  |  |  |  |  |  |  |  |
|  |  |  |  |  |  |  |  |  |
|  |  |  |  |  |  |  |  |  |
|  |  |  |  |  |  |  |  |  |
|  |  |  |  |  |  |  |  |  |
|  |  |  |  |  |  |  |  |  |

| CARDIO: | TIME | DISTANCE | PACE | HR |
|---|---|---|---|---|
|  |  |  |  |  |
|  |  |  |  |  |
|  |  |  |  |  |
|  |  |  |  |  |

| SUPPLEMENTS & VITAMINS | SERVINGS | QUANTITY |
|---|---|---|
|  |  |  |
|  |  |  |
|  |  |  |
|  |  |  |
|  |  |  |

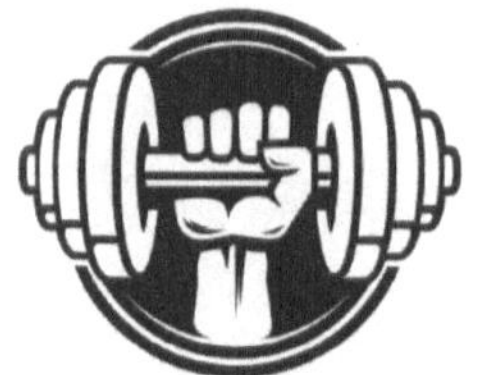

**NAME:** ___________________

**DATE:** ___________________

**TIME START:** ___________________

**TIME END:** ___________________

| WARM-UP | TIME | NOTES |
|---|---|---|
|  |  |  |
|  |  |  |
|  |  |  |
|  |  |  |

| EXERCISE: | SET 1 | | SET 2 | | SET 3 | | SET 4 | |
|---|---|---|---|---|---|---|---|---|
|  | REPS | WEIGHT | REPS | WEIGHT | REPS | WEIGHT | REPS | WEIGHT |
|  |  |  |  |  |  |  |  |  |
|  |  |  |  |  |  |  |  |  |
|  |  |  |  |  |  |  |  |  |
|  |  |  |  |  |  |  |  |  |
|  |  |  |  |  |  |  |  |  |
|  |  |  |  |  |  |  |  |  |
|  |  |  |  |  |  |  |  |  |
|  |  |  |  |  |  |  |  |  |
|  |  |  |  |  |  |  |  |  |
|  |  |  |  |  |  |  |  |  |
|  |  |  |  |  |  |  |  |  |

| CARDIO: | TIME | DISTANCE | PACE | HR |
|---|---|---|---|---|
|  |  |  |  |  |
|  |  |  |  |  |
|  |  |  |  |  |
|  |  |  |  |  |

| SUPPLEMENTS & VITAMINS | SERVINGS | QUANTITY |
|---|---|---|
|  |  |  |
|  |  |  |
|  |  |  |
|  |  |  |
|  |  |  |

NAME:_______________________

DATE:_______________________

TIME START:_______________________

TIME END:_______________________

| WARM-UP | TIME | NOTES |
|---|---|---|
|  |  |  |
|  |  |  |
|  |  |  |
|  |  |  |

| EXERCISE: | SET 1 | | SET 2 | | SET 3 | | SET 4 | |
|---|---|---|---|---|---|---|---|---|
|  | REPS | WEIGHT | REPS | WEIGHT | REPS | WEIGHT | REPS | WEIGHT |
|  |  |  |  |  |  |  |  |  |
|  |  |  |  |  |  |  |  |  |
|  |  |  |  |  |  |  |  |  |
|  |  |  |  |  |  |  |  |  |
|  |  |  |  |  |  |  |  |  |
|  |  |  |  |  |  |  |  |  |
|  |  |  |  |  |  |  |  |  |
|  |  |  |  |  |  |  |  |  |
|  |  |  |  |  |  |  |  |  |
|  |  |  |  |  |  |  |  |  |
|  |  |  |  |  |  |  |  |  |

| CARDIO: | TIME | DISTANCE | PACE | HR |
|---|---|---|---|---|
|  |  |  |  |  |
|  |  |  |  |  |
|  |  |  |  |  |
|  |  |  |  |  |

| SUPPLEMENTS & VITAMINS | SERVINGS | QUANTITY |
|---|---|---|
|  |  |  |
|  |  |  |
|  |  |  |
|  |  |  |
|  |  |  |

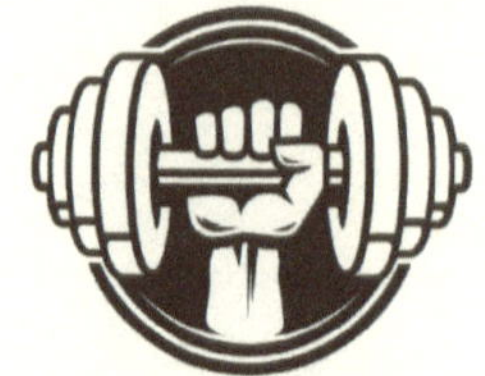

NAME:

DATE:

TIME START:

TIME END:

| WARM-UP | TIME | NOTES |
|---|---|---|
|  |  |  |
|  |  |  |
|  |  |  |
|  |  |  |

| EXERCISE: | SET 1 | | SET 2 | | SET 3 | | SET 4 | |
|---|---|---|---|---|---|---|---|---|
|  | REPS | WEIGHT | REPS | WEIGHT | REPS | WEIGHT | REPS | WEIGHT |
|  |  |  |  |  |  |  |  |  |
|  |  |  |  |  |  |  |  |  |
|  |  |  |  |  |  |  |  |  |
|  |  |  |  |  |  |  |  |  |
|  |  |  |  |  |  |  |  |  |
|  |  |  |  |  |  |  |  |  |
|  |  |  |  |  |  |  |  |  |
|  |  |  |  |  |  |  |  |  |
|  |  |  |  |  |  |  |  |  |
|  |  |  |  |  |  |  |  |  |
|  |  |  |  |  |  |  |  |  |

| CARDIO: | TIME | DISTANCE | PACE | HR |
|---|---|---|---|---|
|  |  |  |  |  |
|  |  |  |  |  |
|  |  |  |  |  |
|  |  |  |  |  |

| SUPPLEMENTS & VITAMINS | SERVINGS | QUANTITY |
|---|---|---|
|  |  |  |
|  |  |  |
|  |  |  |
|  |  |  |

NAME:

DATE:

TIME START:

TIME END:

| WARM-UP | TIME | NOTES |
|---|---|---|
|  |  |  |
|  |  |  |
|  |  |  |
|  |  |  |

| EXERCISE: | SET 1 | | SET 2 | | SET 3 | | SET 4 | |
|---|---|---|---|---|---|---|---|---|
|  | REPS | WEIGHT | REPS | WEIGHT | REPS | WEIGHT | REPS | WEIGHT |
|  |  |  |  |  |  |  |  |  |
|  |  |  |  |  |  |  |  |  |
|  |  |  |  |  |  |  |  |  |
|  |  |  |  |  |  |  |  |  |
|  |  |  |  |  |  |  |  |  |
|  |  |  |  |  |  |  |  |  |
|  |  |  |  |  |  |  |  |  |
|  |  |  |  |  |  |  |  |  |
|  |  |  |  |  |  |  |  |  |
|  |  |  |  |  |  |  |  |  |
|  |  |  |  |  |  |  |  |  |

| CARDIO: | TIME | DISTANCE | PACE | HR |
|---|---|---|---|---|
|  |  |  |  |  |
|  |  |  |  |  |
|  |  |  |  |  |
|  |  |  |  |  |

| SUPPLEMENTS & VITAMINS | SERVINGS | QUANTITY |
|---|---|---|
|  |  |  |
|  |  |  |
|  |  |  |
|  |  |  |
|  |  |  |

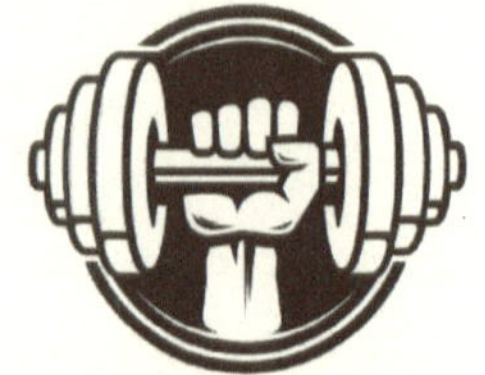

NAME:_______________________________

DATE:_______________________________

TIME START:_________________________

TIME END:___________________________

| WARM-UP | TIME | NOTES |
|---|---|---|
|  |  |  |
|  |  |  |
|  |  |  |
|  |  |  |

| EXERCISE: | SET 1 | | SET 2 | | SET 3 | | SET 4 | |
|---|---|---|---|---|---|---|---|---|
|  | REPS | WEIGHT | REPS | WEIGHT | REPS | WEIGHT | REPS | WEIGHT |
|  |  |  |  |  |  |  |  |  |
|  |  |  |  |  |  |  |  |  |
|  |  |  |  |  |  |  |  |  |
|  |  |  |  |  |  |  |  |  |
|  |  |  |  |  |  |  |  |  |
|  |  |  |  |  |  |  |  |  |
|  |  |  |  |  |  |  |  |  |
|  |  |  |  |  |  |  |  |  |
|  |  |  |  |  |  |  |  |  |
|  |  |  |  |  |  |  |  |  |
|  |  |  |  |  |  |  |  |  |

| CARDIO: | TIME | DISTANCE | PACE | HR |
|---|---|---|---|---|
|  |  |  |  |  |
|  |  |  |  |  |
|  |  |  |  |  |
|  |  |  |  |  |

| SUPPLEMENTS & VITAMINS | SERVINGS | QUANTITY |
|---|---|---|
|  |  |  |
|  |  |  |
|  |  |  |
|  |  |  |

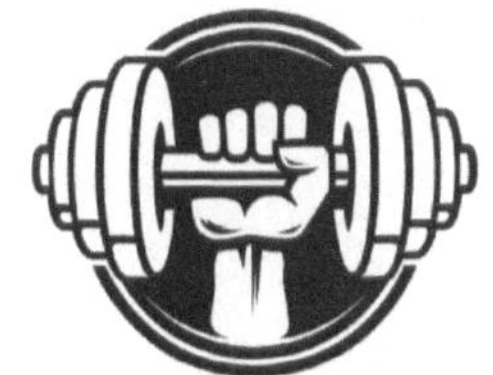

NAME:________________________

DATE:________________________

TIME START:________________________

TIME END:________________________

| WARM-UP | TIME | NOTES |
|---|---|---|
|  |  |  |
|  |  |  |
|  |  |  |
|  |  |  |

| EXERCISE: | SET 1 | | SET 2 | | SET 3 | | SET 4 | |
|---|---|---|---|---|---|---|---|---|
|  | REPS | WEIGHT | REPS | WEIGHT | REPS | WEIGHT | REPS | WEIGHT |
|  |  |  |  |  |  |  |  |  |
|  |  |  |  |  |  |  |  |  |
|  |  |  |  |  |  |  |  |  |
|  |  |  |  |  |  |  |  |  |
|  |  |  |  |  |  |  |  |  |
|  |  |  |  |  |  |  |  |  |
|  |  |  |  |  |  |  |  |  |
|  |  |  |  |  |  |  |  |  |
|  |  |  |  |  |  |  |  |  |
|  |  |  |  |  |  |  |  |  |
|  |  |  |  |  |  |  |  |  |
|  |  |  |  |  |  |  |  |  |

| CARDIO: | TIME | DISTANCE | PACE | HR |
|---|---|---|---|---|
|  |  |  |  |  |
|  |  |  |  |  |
|  |  |  |  |  |
|  |  |  |  |  |

| SUPPLEMENTS & VITAMINS | SERVINGS | QUANTITY |
|---|---|---|
|  |  |  |
|  |  |  |
|  |  |  |
|  |  |  |
|  |  |  |

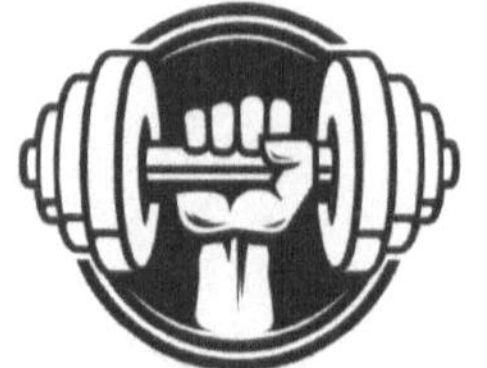

NAME:_______________________________

DATE:_______________________________

TIME START:_______________________________

TIME END:_______________________________

| WARM-UP | TIME | NOTES |
|---------|------|-------|
|  |  |  |
|  |  |  |
|  |  |  |
|  |  |  |

| EXERCISE: | SET 1 | | SET 2 | | SET 3 | | SET 4 | |
|-----------|-------|--------|-------|--------|-------|--------|-------|--------|
|  | REPS | WEIGHT | REPS | WEIGHT | REPS | WEIGHT | REPS | WEIGHT |
|  |  |  |  |  |  |  |  |  |
|  |  |  |  |  |  |  |  |  |
|  |  |  |  |  |  |  |  |  |
|  |  |  |  |  |  |  |  |  |
|  |  |  |  |  |  |  |  |  |
|  |  |  |  |  |  |  |  |  |
|  |  |  |  |  |  |  |  |  |
|  |  |  |  |  |  |  |  |  |
|  |  |  |  |  |  |  |  |  |
|  |  |  |  |  |  |  |  |  |
|  |  |  |  |  |  |  |  |  |

| CARDIO: | TIME | DISTANCE | PACE | HR |
|---------|------|----------|------|----|
|  |  |  |  |  |
|  |  |  |  |  |
|  |  |  |  |  |
|  |  |  |  |  |

| SUPPLEMENTS & VITAMINS | SERVINGS | QUANTITY |
|------------------------|----------|----------|
|  |  |  |
|  |  |  |
|  |  |  |
|  |  |  |
|  |  |  |

NAME: ___________________

DATE: ___________________

TIME START: ___________________

TIME END: ___________________

| WARM-UP | TIME | NOTES |
|---|---|---|
|  |  |  |
|  |  |  |
|  |  |  |
|  |  |  |

| EXERCISE: | SET 1 | | SET 2 | | SET 3 | | SET 4 | |
|---|---|---|---|---|---|---|---|---|
|  | REPS | WEIGHT | REPS | WEIGHT | REPS | WEIGHT | REPS | WEIGHT |
|  |  |  |  |  |  |  |  |  |
|  |  |  |  |  |  |  |  |  |
|  |  |  |  |  |  |  |  |  |
|  |  |  |  |  |  |  |  |  |
|  |  |  |  |  |  |  |  |  |
|  |  |  |  |  |  |  |  |  |
|  |  |  |  |  |  |  |  |  |
|  |  |  |  |  |  |  |  |  |
|  |  |  |  |  |  |  |  |  |
|  |  |  |  |  |  |  |  |  |
|  |  |  |  |  |  |  |  |  |
|  |  |  |  |  |  |  |  |  |

| CARDIO: | TIME | DISTANCE | PACE | HR |
|---|---|---|---|---|
|  |  |  |  |  |
|  |  |  |  |  |
|  |  |  |  |  |
|  |  |  |  |  |

| SUPPLEMENTS & VITAMINS | SERVINGS | QUANTITY |
|---|---|---|
|  |  |  |
|  |  |  |
|  |  |  |
|  |  |  |

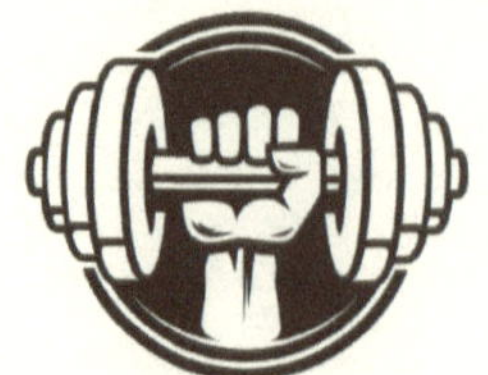

NAME:

DATE:

TIME START:

TIME END:

| WARM-UP | TIME | NOTES |
| --- | --- | --- |
|  |  |  |
|  |  |  |
|  |  |  |

| EXERCISE: | SET 1 | | SET 2 | | SET 3 | | SET 4 | |
| --- | --- | --- | --- | --- | --- | --- | --- | --- |
|  | REPS | WEIGHT | REPS | WEIGHT | REPS | WEIGHT | REPS | WEIGHT |
|  |  |  |  |  |  |  |  |  |
|  |  |  |  |  |  |  |  |  |
|  |  |  |  |  |  |  |  |  |
|  |  |  |  |  |  |  |  |  |
|  |  |  |  |  |  |  |  |  |
|  |  |  |  |  |  |  |  |  |
|  |  |  |  |  |  |  |  |  |

| CARDIO: | TIME | DISTANCE | PACE | HR |
| --- | --- | --- | --- | --- |
|  |  |  |  |  |
|  |  |  |  |  |
|  |  |  |  |  |

| SUPPLEMENTS & VITAMINS | SERVINGS | QUANTITY |
| --- | --- | --- |
|  |  |  |
|  |  |  |
|  |  |  |

NAME:_______________________________

DATE:_______________________________

TIME START:_______________________________

TIME END:_______________________________

| WARM-UP | TIME | NOTES |
|---|---|---|
| | | |
| | | |
| | | |

| EXERCISE: | SET 1 | | SET 2 | | SET 3 | | SET 4 | |
|---|---|---|---|---|---|---|---|---|
| | REPS | WEIGHT | REPS | WEIGHT | REPS | WEIGHT | REPS | WEIGHT |
| | | | | | | | | |
| | | | | | | | | |
| | | | | | | | | |
| | | | | | | | | |
| | | | | | | | | |
| | | | | | | | | |
| | | | | | | | | |
| | | | | | | | | |
| | | | | | | | | |
| | | | | | | | | |

| CARDIO: | TIME | DISTANCE | PACE | HR |
|---|---|---|---|---|
| | | | | |
| | | | | |
| | | | | |

| SUPPLEMENTS & VITAMINS | SERVINGS | QUANTITY |
|---|---|---|
| | | |
| | | |
| | | |
| | | |

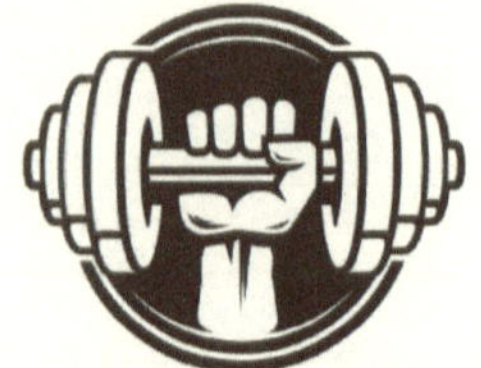

NAME:

DATE:

TIME START:

TIME END:

| WARM-UP | TIME | NOTES |
|---|---|---|
|  |  |  |
|  |  |  |
|  |  |  |
|  |  |  |

| EXERCISE: | SET 1 | | SET 2 | | SET 3 | | SET 4 | |
|---|---|---|---|---|---|---|---|---|
|  | REPS | WEIGHT | REPS | WEIGHT | REPS | WEIGHT | REPS | WEIGHT |
|  |  |  |  |  |  |  |  |  |
|  |  |  |  |  |  |  |  |  |
|  |  |  |  |  |  |  |  |  |
|  |  |  |  |  |  |  |  |  |
|  |  |  |  |  |  |  |  |  |
|  |  |  |  |  |  |  |  |  |
|  |  |  |  |  |  |  |  |  |
|  |  |  |  |  |  |  |  |  |
|  |  |  |  |  |  |  |  |  |
|  |  |  |  |  |  |  |  |  |
|  |  |  |  |  |  |  |  |  |
|  |  |  |  |  |  |  |  |  |

| CARDIO: | TIME | DISTANCE | PACE | HR |
|---|---|---|---|---|
|  |  |  |  |  |
|  |  |  |  |  |
|  |  |  |  |  |
|  |  |  |  |  |

| SUPPLEMENTS & VITAMINS | SERVINGS | QUANTITY |
|---|---|---|
|  |  |  |
|  |  |  |
|  |  |  |
|  |  |  |
|  |  |  |

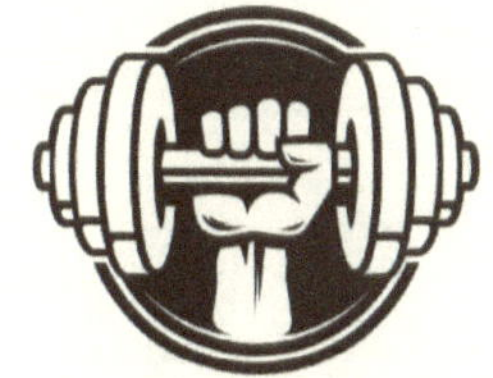

**NAME:**_______________________

**DATE:**_______________________

**TIME START:**_______________________

**TIME END:**_______________________

| WARM-UP | TIME | NOTES |
|---|---|---|
| | | |
| | | |
| | | |
| | | |

| EXERCISE: | SET 1 | | SET 2 | | SET 3 | | SET 4 | |
|---|---|---|---|---|---|---|---|---|
| | REPS | WEIGHT | REPS | WEIGHT | REPS | WEIGHT | REPS | WEIGHT |
| | | | | | | | | |
| | | | | | | | | |
| | | | | | | | | |
| | | | | | | | | |
| | | | | | | | | |
| | | | | | | | | |
| | | | | | | | | |
| | | | | | | | | |
| | | | | | | | | |
| | | | | | | | | |
| | | | | | | | | |

| CARDIO: | TIME | DISTANCE | PACE | HR |
|---|---|---|---|---|
| | | | | |
| | | | | |
| | | | | |
| | | | | |

| SUPPLEMENTS & VITAMINS | SERVINGS | QUANTITY |
|---|---|---|
| | | |
| | | |
| | | |
| | | |
| | | |

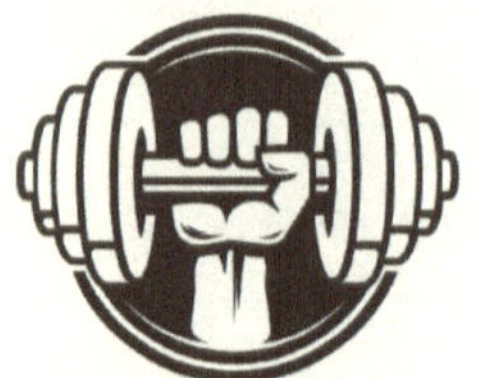

NAME:

DATE:

TIME START:

TIME END:

| WARM-UP | TIME | NOTES |
|---|---|---|
|  |  |  |
|  |  |  |
|  |  |  |
|  |  |  |

| EXERCISE: | SET 1 | | SET 2 | | SET 3 | | SET 4 | |
|---|---|---|---|---|---|---|---|---|
|  | REPS | WEIGHT | REPS | WEIGHT | REPS | WEIGHT | REPS | WEIGHT |
|  |  |  |  |  |  |  |  |  |
|  |  |  |  |  |  |  |  |  |
|  |  |  |  |  |  |  |  |  |
|  |  |  |  |  |  |  |  |  |
|  |  |  |  |  |  |  |  |  |
|  |  |  |  |  |  |  |  |  |
|  |  |  |  |  |  |  |  |  |
|  |  |  |  |  |  |  |  |  |
|  |  |  |  |  |  |  |  |  |
|  |  |  |  |  |  |  |  |  |
|  |  |  |  |  |  |  |  |  |

| CARDIO: | TIME | DISTANCE | PACE | HR |
|---|---|---|---|---|
|  |  |  |  |  |
|  |  |  |  |  |
|  |  |  |  |  |
|  |  |  |  |  |

| SUPPLEMENTS & VITAMINS | SERVINGS | QUANTITY |
|---|---|---|
|  |  |  |
|  |  |  |
|  |  |  |
|  |  |  |

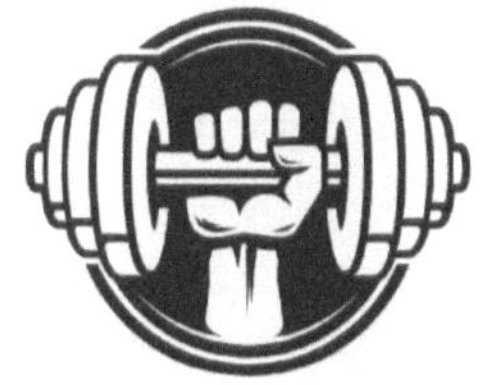

NAME:_______________________

DATE:_______________________

TIME START:_______________________

TIME END:_______________________

| WARM-UP | TIME | NOTES |
|---------|------|-------|
|  |  |  |
|  |  |  |
|  |  |  |
|  |  |  |

| EXERCISE: | SET 1 | | SET 2 | | SET 3 | | SET 4 | |
|-----------|-------|--------|-------|--------|-------|--------|-------|--------|
|  | REPS | WEIGHT | REPS | WEIGHT | REPS | WEIGHT | REPS | WEIGHT |
|  |  |  |  |  |  |  |  |  |
|  |  |  |  |  |  |  |  |  |
|  |  |  |  |  |  |  |  |  |
|  |  |  |  |  |  |  |  |  |
|  |  |  |  |  |  |  |  |  |
|  |  |  |  |  |  |  |  |  |
|  |  |  |  |  |  |  |  |  |
|  |  |  |  |  |  |  |  |  |
|  |  |  |  |  |  |  |  |  |
|  |  |  |  |  |  |  |  |  |
|  |  |  |  |  |  |  |  |  |

| CARDIO: | TIME | DISTANCE | PACE | HR |
|---------|------|----------|------|-----|
|  |  |  |  |  |
|  |  |  |  |  |
|  |  |  |  |  |
|  |  |  |  |  |

| SUPPLEMENTS & VITAMINS | SERVINGS | QUANTITY |
|------------------------|----------|----------|
|  |  |  |
|  |  |  |
|  |  |  |
|  |  |  |
|  |  |  |

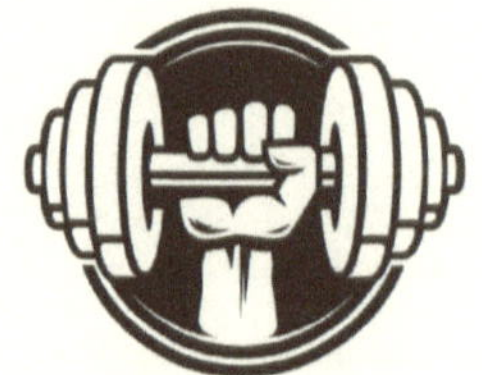

NAME:______________________________

DATE:______________________________

TIME START:______________________________

TIME END:______________________________

| WARM-UP | TIME | NOTES |
|---|---|---|
|  |  |  |
|  |  |  |
|  |  |  |
|  |  |  |

| EXERCISE: | SET 1 | | SET 2 | | SET 3 | | SET 4 | |
|---|---|---|---|---|---|---|---|---|
|  | REPS | WEIGHT | REPS | WEIGHT | REPS | WEIGHT | REPS | WEIGHT |
|  |  |  |  |  |  |  |  |  |
|  |  |  |  |  |  |  |  |  |
|  |  |  |  |  |  |  |  |  |
|  |  |  |  |  |  |  |  |  |
|  |  |  |  |  |  |  |  |  |
|  |  |  |  |  |  |  |  |  |
|  |  |  |  |  |  |  |  |  |
|  |  |  |  |  |  |  |  |  |
|  |  |  |  |  |  |  |  |  |
|  |  |  |  |  |  |  |  |  |

| CARDIO: | TIME | DISTANCE | PACE | HR |
|---|---|---|---|---|
|  |  |  |  |  |
|  |  |  |  |  |
|  |  |  |  |  |
|  |  |  |  |  |

| SUPPLEMENTS & VITAMINS | SERVINGS | QUANTITY |
|---|---|---|
|  |  |  |
|  |  |  |
|  |  |  |
|  |  |  |

NAME:_______________________________

DATE:_______________________________

TIME START:_________________________

TIME END:___________________________

| WARM-UP | TIME | NOTES |
|---|---|---|
|  |  |  |
|  |  |  |
|  |  |  |
|  |  |  |

| EXERCISE: | SET 1 | | SET 2 | | SET 3 | | SET 4 | |
|---|---|---|---|---|---|---|---|---|
|  | REPS | WEIGHT | REPS | WEIGHT | REPS | WEIGHT | REPS | WEIGHT |
|  |  |  |  |  |  |  |  |  |
|  |  |  |  |  |  |  |  |  |
|  |  |  |  |  |  |  |  |  |
|  |  |  |  |  |  |  |  |  |
|  |  |  |  |  |  |  |  |  |
|  |  |  |  |  |  |  |  |  |
|  |  |  |  |  |  |  |  |  |
|  |  |  |  |  |  |  |  |  |
|  |  |  |  |  |  |  |  |  |
|  |  |  |  |  |  |  |  |  |
|  |  |  |  |  |  |  |  |  |

| CARDIO: | TIME | DISTANCE | PACE | HR |
|---|---|---|---|---|
|  |  |  |  |  |
|  |  |  |  |  |
|  |  |  |  |  |
|  |  |  |  |  |

| SUPPLEMENTS & VITAMINS | SERVINGS | QUANTITY |
|---|---|---|
|  |  |  |
|  |  |  |
|  |  |  |
|  |  |  |
|  |  |  |

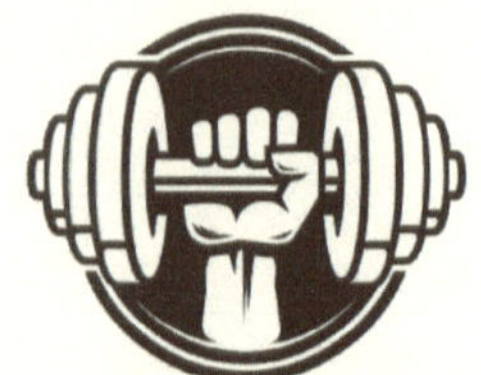

NAME:_______________________________

DATE:_______________________________

TIME START:_________________________

TIME END:___________________________

| WARM-UP | TIME | NOTES |
|---|---|---|
| | | |
| | | |
| | | |
| | | |

| EXERCISE: | SET 1 | | SET 2 | | SET 3 | | SET 4 | |
|---|---|---|---|---|---|---|---|---|
| | REPS | WEIGHT | REPS | WEIGHT | REPS | WEIGHT | REPS | WEIGHT |
| | | | | | | | | |
| | | | | | | | | |
| | | | | | | | | |
| | | | | | | | | |
| | | | | | | | | |
| | | | | | | | | |
| | | | | | | | | |
| | | | | | | | | |
| | | | | | | | | |
| | | | | | | | | |
| | | | | | | | | |

| CARDIO: | TIME | DISTANCE | PACE | HR |
|---|---|---|---|---|
| | | | | |
| | | | | |
| | | | | |
| | | | | |

| SUPPLEMENTS & VITAMINS | SERVINGS | QUANTITY |
|---|---|---|
| | | |
| | | |
| | | |
| | | |
| | | |

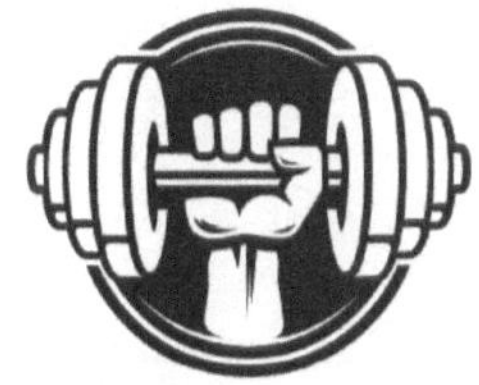

NAME:_____________________________

DATE:_____________________________

TIME START:_____________________________

TIME END:_____________________________

| WARM-UP | TIME | NOTES |
|---|---|---|
| | | |
| | | |
| | | |
| | | |

| EXERCISE: | SET 1 | | SET 2 | | SET 3 | | SET 4 | |
|---|---|---|---|---|---|---|---|---|
| | REPS | WEIGHT | REPS | WEIGHT | REPS | WEIGHT | REPS | WEIGHT |
| | | | | | | | | |
| | | | | | | | | |
| | | | | | | | | |
| | | | | | | | | |
| | | | | | | | | |
| | | | | | | | | |
| | | | | | | | | |
| | | | | | | | | |
| | | | | | | | | |
| | | | | | | | | |
| | | | | | | | | |

| CARDIO: | TIME | DISTANCE | PACE | HR |
|---|---|---|---|---|
| | | | | |
| | | | | |
| | | | | |
| | | | | |

| SUPPLEMENTS & VITAMINS | SERVINGS | QUANTITY |
|---|---|---|
| | | |
| | | |
| | | |
| | | |
| | | |

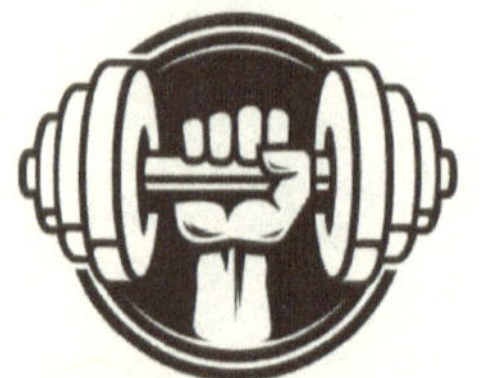

NAME:

DATE:

TIME START:

TIME END:

| WARM-UP | TIME | NOTES |
|---|---|---|
|  |  |  |
|  |  |  |
|  |  |  |
|  |  |  |

| EXERCISE: | SET 1 | | SET 2 | | SET 3 | | SET 4 | |
|---|---|---|---|---|---|---|---|---|
|  | REPS | WEIGHT | REPS | WEIGHT | REPS | WEIGHT | REPS | WEIGHT |
|  |  |  |  |  |  |  |  |  |
|  |  |  |  |  |  |  |  |  |
|  |  |  |  |  |  |  |  |  |
|  |  |  |  |  |  |  |  |  |
|  |  |  |  |  |  |  |  |  |
|  |  |  |  |  |  |  |  |  |
|  |  |  |  |  |  |  |  |  |
|  |  |  |  |  |  |  |  |  |
|  |  |  |  |  |  |  |  |  |
|  |  |  |  |  |  |  |  |  |
|  |  |  |  |  |  |  |  |  |

| CARDIO: | TIME | DISTANCE | PACE | HR |
|---|---|---|---|---|
|  |  |  |  |  |
|  |  |  |  |  |
|  |  |  |  |  |
|  |  |  |  |  |

| SUPPLEMENTS & VITAMINS | SERVINGS | QUANTITY |
|---|---|---|
|  |  |  |
|  |  |  |
|  |  |  |
|  |  |  |
|  |  |  |

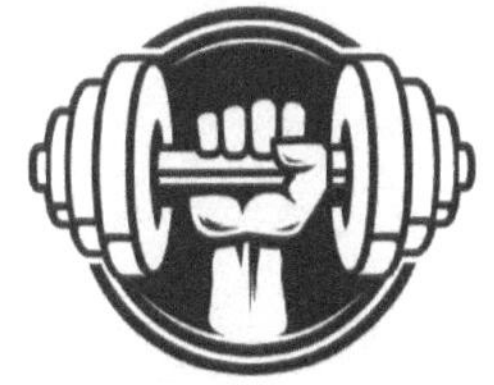

NAME:_______________________

DATE:_______________________

TIME START:_______________________

TIME END:_______________________

| WARM-UP | TIME | NOTES |
|---------|------|-------|
|  |  |  |
|  |  |  |
|  |  |  |
|  |  |  |

| EXERCISE: | SET 1 | | SET 2 | | SET 3 | | SET 4 | |
|-----------|-------|--------|-------|--------|-------|--------|-------|--------|
|  | REPS | WEIGHT | REPS | WEIGHT | REPS | WEIGHT | REPS | WEIGHT |
|  |  |  |  |  |  |  |  |  |
|  |  |  |  |  |  |  |  |  |
|  |  |  |  |  |  |  |  |  |
|  |  |  |  |  |  |  |  |  |
|  |  |  |  |  |  |  |  |  |
|  |  |  |  |  |  |  |  |  |
|  |  |  |  |  |  |  |  |  |
|  |  |  |  |  |  |  |  |  |
|  |  |  |  |  |  |  |  |  |
|  |  |  |  |  |  |  |  |  |
|  |  |  |  |  |  |  |  |  |

| CARDIO: | TIME | DISTANCE | PACE | HR |
|---------|------|----------|------|-----|
|  |  |  |  |  |
|  |  |  |  |  |
|  |  |  |  |  |
|  |  |  |  |  |

| SUPPLEMENTS & VITAMINS | SERVINGS | QUANTITY |
|------------------------|----------|----------|
|  |  |  |
|  |  |  |
|  |  |  |
|  |  |  |
|  |  |  |

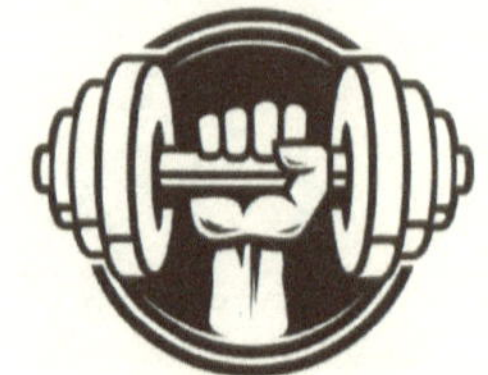

NAME:

DATE:

TIME START:

TIME END:

| WARM-UP | TIME | NOTES |
|---|---|---|
|  |  |  |
|  |  |  |
|  |  |  |
|  |  |  |

| EXERCISE: | SET 1 | | SET 2 | | SET 3 | | SET 4 | |
|---|---|---|---|---|---|---|---|---|
|  | REPS | WEIGHT | REPS | WEIGHT | REPS | WEIGHT | REPS | WEIGHT |
|  |  |  |  |  |  |  |  |  |
|  |  |  |  |  |  |  |  |  |
|  |  |  |  |  |  |  |  |  |
|  |  |  |  |  |  |  |  |  |
|  |  |  |  |  |  |  |  |  |
|  |  |  |  |  |  |  |  |  |
|  |  |  |  |  |  |  |  |  |
|  |  |  |  |  |  |  |  |  |
|  |  |  |  |  |  |  |  |  |
|  |  |  |  |  |  |  |  |  |
|  |  |  |  |  |  |  |  |  |
|  |  |  |  |  |  |  |  |  |

| CARDIO: | TIME | DISTANCE | PACE | HR |
|---|---|---|---|---|
|  |  |  |  |  |
|  |  |  |  |  |
|  |  |  |  |  |
|  |  |  |  |  |

| SUPPLEMENTS & VITAMINS | SERVINGS | QUANTITY |
|---|---|---|
|  |  |  |
|  |  |  |
|  |  |  |
|  |  |  |

NAME:_______________________________

DATE:_______________________________

TIME START:_______________________________

TIME END:_______________________________

| WARM-UP | TIME | NOTES |
|---------|------|-------|
|  |  |  |
|  |  |  |
|  |  |  |
|  |  |  |

| EXERCISE: | SET 1 | | SET 2 | | SET 3 | | SET 4 | |
|-----------|-------|--------|-------|--------|-------|--------|-------|--------|
|  | REPS | WEIGHT | REPS | WEIGHT | REPS | WEIGHT | REPS | WEIGHT |
|  |  |  |  |  |  |  |  |  |
|  |  |  |  |  |  |  |  |  |
|  |  |  |  |  |  |  |  |  |
|  |  |  |  |  |  |  |  |  |
|  |  |  |  |  |  |  |  |  |
|  |  |  |  |  |  |  |  |  |
|  |  |  |  |  |  |  |  |  |
|  |  |  |  |  |  |  |  |  |
|  |  |  |  |  |  |  |  |  |
|  |  |  |  |  |  |  |  |  |
|  |  |  |  |  |  |  |  |  |
|  |  |  |  |  |  |  |  |  |

| CARDIO: | TIME | DISTANCE | PACE | HR |
|---------|------|----------|------|-----|
|  |  |  |  |  |
|  |  |  |  |  |
|  |  |  |  |  |
|  |  |  |  |  |

| SUPPLEMENTS & VITAMINS | SERVINGS | QUANTITY |
|------------------------|----------|----------|
|  |  |  |
|  |  |  |
|  |  |  |
|  |  |  |
|  |  |  |

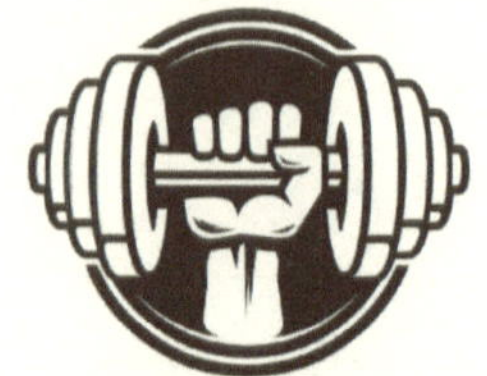

NAME:

DATE:

TIME START:

TIME END:

| WARM-UP | TIME | NOTES |
|---|---|---|
|  |  |  |
|  |  |  |
|  |  |  |
|  |  |  |

| EXERCISE: | SET 1 | | SET 2 | | SET 3 | | SET 4 | |
|---|---|---|---|---|---|---|---|---|
|  | REPS | WEIGHT | REPS | WEIGHT | REPS | WEIGHT | REPS | WEIGHT |
|  |  |  |  |  |  |  |  |  |
|  |  |  |  |  |  |  |  |  |
|  |  |  |  |  |  |  |  |  |
|  |  |  |  |  |  |  |  |  |
|  |  |  |  |  |  |  |  |  |
|  |  |  |  |  |  |  |  |  |
|  |  |  |  |  |  |  |  |  |
|  |  |  |  |  |  |  |  |  |
|  |  |  |  |  |  |  |  |  |
|  |  |  |  |  |  |  |  |  |
|  |  |  |  |  |  |  |  |  |

| CARDIO: | TIME | DISTANCE | PACE | HR |
|---|---|---|---|---|
|  |  |  |  |  |
|  |  |  |  |  |
|  |  |  |  |  |
|  |  |  |  |  |

| SUPPLEMENTS & VITAMINS | SERVINGS | QUANTITY |
|---|---|---|
|  |  |  |
|  |  |  |
|  |  |  |
|  |  |  |

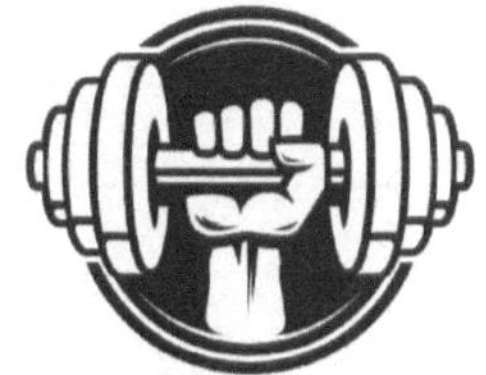

NAME:_______________________________

DATE:_______________________________

TIME START:_______________________________

TIME END:_______________________________

| WARM-UP | TIME | NOTES |
|---|---|---|
|  |  |  |
|  |  |  |
|  |  |  |
|  |  |  |

| EXERCISE: | SET 1 | | SET 2 | | SET 3 | | SET 4 | |
|---|---|---|---|---|---|---|---|---|
|  | REPS | WEIGHT | REPS | WEIGHT | REPS | WEIGHT | REPS | WEIGHT |
|  |  |  |  |  |  |  |  |  |
|  |  |  |  |  |  |  |  |  |
|  |  |  |  |  |  |  |  |  |
|  |  |  |  |  |  |  |  |  |
|  |  |  |  |  |  |  |  |  |
|  |  |  |  |  |  |  |  |  |
|  |  |  |  |  |  |  |  |  |
|  |  |  |  |  |  |  |  |  |
|  |  |  |  |  |  |  |  |  |
|  |  |  |  |  |  |  |  |  |
|  |  |  |  |  |  |  |  |  |
|  |  |  |  |  |  |  |  |  |

| CARDIO: | TIME | DISTANCE | PACE | HR |
|---|---|---|---|---|
|  |  |  |  |  |
|  |  |  |  |  |
|  |  |  |  |  |
|  |  |  |  |  |

| SUPPLEMENTS & VITAMINS | SERVINGS | QUANTITY |
|---|---|---|
|  |  |  |
|  |  |  |
|  |  |  |
|  |  |  |
|  |  |  |

NAME:_______________________________

DATE:_______________________________

TIME START:_______________________________

TIME END:_______________________________

| WARM-UP | TIME | NOTES |
|---|---|---|
| | | |
| | | |
| | | |
| | | |

| EXERCISE: | SET 1 | | SET 2 | | SET 3 | | SET 4 | |
|---|---|---|---|---|---|---|---|---|
| | REPS | WEIGHT | REPS | WEIGHT | REPS | WEIGHT | REPS | WEIGHT |
| | | | | | | | | |
| | | | | | | | | |
| | | | | | | | | |
| | | | | | | | | |
| | | | | | | | | |
| | | | | | | | | |
| | | | | | | | | |
| | | | | | | | | |
| | | | | | | | | |
| | | | | | | | | |

| CARDIO: | TIME | DISTANCE | PACE | HR |
|---|---|---|---|---|
| | | | | |
| | | | | |
| | | | | |
| | | | | |

| SUPPLEMENTS & VITAMINS | SERVINGS | QUANTITY |
|---|---|---|
| | | |
| | | |
| | | |
| | | |

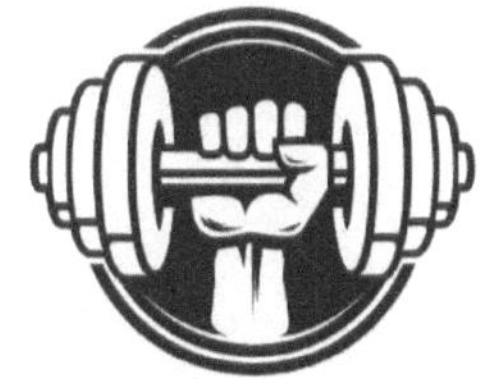

NAME:______________________________

DATE:______________________________

TIME START:______________________________

TIME END:______________________________

| WARM-UP | TIME | NOTES |
|---------|------|-------|
|  |  |  |
|  |  |  |
|  |  |  |
|  |  |  |

| EXERCISE: | SET 1 | | SET 2 | | SET 3 | | SET 4 | |
|-----------|-------|--------|-------|--------|-------|--------|-------|--------|
|  | REPS | WEIGHT | REPS | WEIGHT | REPS | WEIGHT | REPS | WEIGHT |
|  |  |  |  |  |  |  |  |  |
|  |  |  |  |  |  |  |  |  |
|  |  |  |  |  |  |  |  |  |
|  |  |  |  |  |  |  |  |  |
|  |  |  |  |  |  |  |  |  |
|  |  |  |  |  |  |  |  |  |
|  |  |  |  |  |  |  |  |  |
|  |  |  |  |  |  |  |  |  |
|  |  |  |  |  |  |  |  |  |
|  |  |  |  |  |  |  |  |  |

| CARDIO: | TIME | DISTANCE | PACE | HR |
|---------|------|----------|------|----|
|  |  |  |  |  |
|  |  |  |  |  |
|  |  |  |  |  |
|  |  |  |  |  |

| SUPPLEMENTS & VITAMINS | SERVINGS | QUANTITY |
|------------------------|----------|----------|
|  |  |  |
|  |  |  |
|  |  |  |
|  |  |  |
|  |  |  |

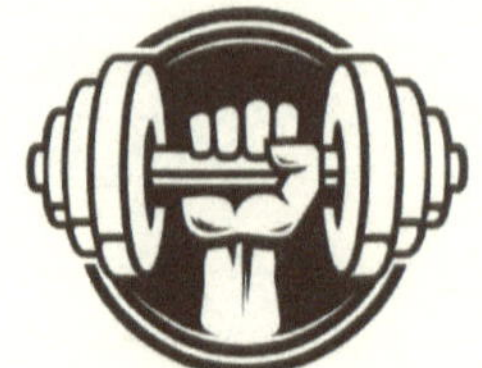

NAME:

DATE:

TIME START:

TIME END:

| WARM-UP | TIME | NOTES |
|---|---|---|
|  |  |  |
|  |  |  |
|  |  |  |
|  |  |  |

| EXERCISE: | SET 1 | | SET 2 | | SET 3 | | SET 4 | |
|---|---|---|---|---|---|---|---|---|
|  | REPS | WEIGHT | REPS | WEIGHT | REPS | WEIGHT | REPS | WEIGHT |
|  |  |  |  |  |  |  |  |  |
|  |  |  |  |  |  |  |  |  |
|  |  |  |  |  |  |  |  |  |
|  |  |  |  |  |  |  |  |  |
|  |  |  |  |  |  |  |  |  |
|  |  |  |  |  |  |  |  |  |
|  |  |  |  |  |  |  |  |  |
|  |  |  |  |  |  |  |  |  |
|  |  |  |  |  |  |  |  |  |
|  |  |  |  |  |  |  |  |  |
|  |  |  |  |  |  |  |  |  |
|  |  |  |  |  |  |  |  |  |

| CARDIO: | TIME | DISTANCE | PACE | HR |
|---|---|---|---|---|
|  |  |  |  |  |
|  |  |  |  |  |
|  |  |  |  |  |
|  |  |  |  |  |

| SUPPLEMENTS & VITAMINS | SERVINGS | QUANTITY |
|---|---|---|
|  |  |  |
|  |  |  |
|  |  |  |
|  |  |  |

NAME:________________________________

DATE:________________________________

TIME START:________________________________

TIME END:________________________________

| WARM-UP | TIME | NOTES |
|---|---|---|
| | | |
| | | |
| | | |
| | | |

| EXERCISE: | SET 1 | | SET 2 | | SET 3 | | SET 4 | |
|---|---|---|---|---|---|---|---|---|
| | REPS | WEIGHT | REPS | WEIGHT | REPS | WEIGHT | REPS | WEIGHT |
| | | | | | | | | |
| | | | | | | | | |
| | | | | | | | | |
| | | | | | | | | |
| | | | | | | | | |
| | | | | | | | | |
| | | | | | | | | |
| | | | | | | | | |
| | | | | | | | | |
| | | | | | | | | |

| CARDIO: | TIME | DISTANCE | PACE | HR |
|---|---|---|---|---|
| | | | | |
| | | | | |
| | | | | |
| | | | | |

| SUPPLEMENTS & VITAMINS | SERVINGS | QUANTITY |
|---|---|---|
| | | |
| | | |
| | | |
| | | |
| | | |

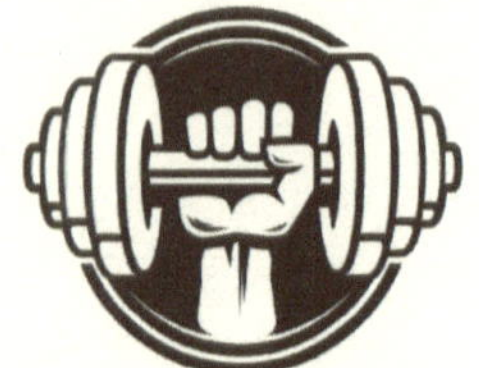

NAME:_______________________________

DATE:_______________________________

TIME START:_________________________

TIME END:___________________________

| WARM-UP | TIME | NOTES |
|---|---|---|
|  |  |  |
|  |  |  |
|  |  |  |
|  |  |  |

| EXERCISE: | SET 1 | | SET 2 | | SET 3 | | SET 4 | |
|---|---|---|---|---|---|---|---|---|
|  | REPS | WEIGHT | REPS | WEIGHT | REPS | WEIGHT | REPS | WEIGHT |
|  |  |  |  |  |  |  |  |  |
|  |  |  |  |  |  |  |  |  |
|  |  |  |  |  |  |  |  |  |
|  |  |  |  |  |  |  |  |  |
|  |  |  |  |  |  |  |  |  |
|  |  |  |  |  |  |  |  |  |
|  |  |  |  |  |  |  |  |  |
|  |  |  |  |  |  |  |  |  |
|  |  |  |  |  |  |  |  |  |
|  |  |  |  |  |  |  |  |  |
|  |  |  |  |  |  |  |  |  |

| CARDIO: | TIME | DISTANCE | PACE | HR |
|---|---|---|---|---|
|  |  |  |  |  |
|  |  |  |  |  |
|  |  |  |  |  |
|  |  |  |  |  |

| SUPPLEMENTS & VITAMINS | SERVINGS | QUANTITY |
|---|---|---|
|  |  |  |
|  |  |  |
|  |  |  |
|  |  |  |
|  |  |  |

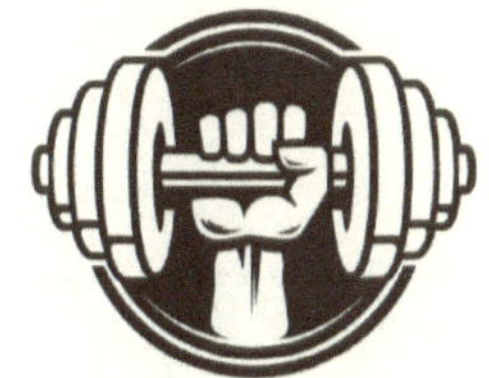

NAME:________________________________

DATE:________________________________

TIME START:________________________________

TIME END:________________________________

| WARM-UP | TIME | NOTES |
|---|---|---|
|  |  |  |
|  |  |  |
|  |  |  |
|  |  |  |

| EXERCISE: | SET 1 | | SET 2 | | SET 3 | | SET 4 | |
|---|---|---|---|---|---|---|---|---|
|  | REPS | WEIGHT | REPS | WEIGHT | REPS | WEIGHT | REPS | WEIGHT |
|  |  |  |  |  |  |  |  |  |
|  |  |  |  |  |  |  |  |  |
|  |  |  |  |  |  |  |  |  |
|  |  |  |  |  |  |  |  |  |
|  |  |  |  |  |  |  |  |  |
|  |  |  |  |  |  |  |  |  |
|  |  |  |  |  |  |  |  |  |
|  |  |  |  |  |  |  |  |  |
|  |  |  |  |  |  |  |  |  |
|  |  |  |  |  |  |  |  |  |
|  |  |  |  |  |  |  |  |  |
|  |  |  |  |  |  |  |  |  |

| CARDIO: | TIME | DISTANCE | PACE | HR |
|---|---|---|---|---|
|  |  |  |  |  |
|  |  |  |  |  |
|  |  |  |  |  |
|  |  |  |  |  |

| SUPPLEMENTS & VITAMINS | SERVINGS | QUANTITY |
|---|---|---|
|  |  |  |
|  |  |  |
|  |  |  |
|  |  |  |
|  |  |  |

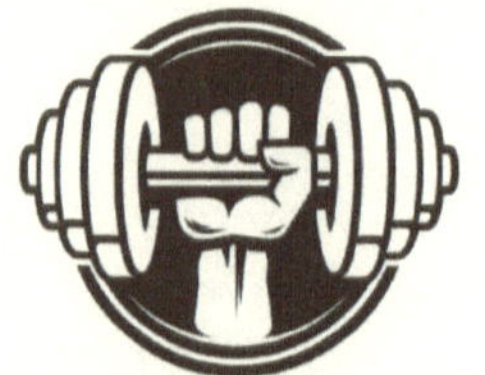

NAME:

DATE:

TIME START:

TIME END:

| WARM-UP | TIME | NOTES |
|---|---|---|
|  |  |  |
|  |  |  |
|  |  |  |
|  |  |  |

| EXERCISE: | SET 1 | | SET 2 | | SET 3 | | SET 4 | |
|---|---|---|---|---|---|---|---|---|
|  | REPS | WEIGHT | REPS | WEIGHT | REPS | WEIGHT | REPS | WEIGHT |
|  |  |  |  |  |  |  |  |  |
|  |  |  |  |  |  |  |  |  |
|  |  |  |  |  |  |  |  |  |
|  |  |  |  |  |  |  |  |  |
|  |  |  |  |  |  |  |  |  |
|  |  |  |  |  |  |  |  |  |
|  |  |  |  |  |  |  |  |  |
|  |  |  |  |  |  |  |  |  |
|  |  |  |  |  |  |  |  |  |
|  |  |  |  |  |  |  |  |  |
|  |  |  |  |  |  |  |  |  |
|  |  |  |  |  |  |  |  |  |

| CARDIO: | TIME | DISTANCE | PACE | HR |
|---|---|---|---|---|
|  |  |  |  |  |
|  |  |  |  |  |
|  |  |  |  |  |
|  |  |  |  |  |

| SUPPLEMENTS & VITAMINS | SERVINGS | QUANTITY |
|---|---|---|
|  |  |  |
|  |  |  |
|  |  |  |
|  |  |  |

NAME:________________________________

DATE:________________________________

TIME START:________________________________

TIME END:________________________________

| WARM-UP | TIME | NOTES |
|---|---|---|
|  |  |  |
|  |  |  |
|  |  |  |
|  |  |  |

| EXERCISE: | SET 1 | | SET 2 | | SET 3 | | SET 4 | |
|---|---|---|---|---|---|---|---|---|
|  | REPS | WEIGHT | REPS | WEIGHT | REPS | WEIGHT | REPS | WEIGHT |
|  |  |  |  |  |  |  |  |  |
|  |  |  |  |  |  |  |  |  |
|  |  |  |  |  |  |  |  |  |
|  |  |  |  |  |  |  |  |  |
|  |  |  |  |  |  |  |  |  |
|  |  |  |  |  |  |  |  |  |
|  |  |  |  |  |  |  |  |  |
|  |  |  |  |  |  |  |  |  |
|  |  |  |  |  |  |  |  |  |
|  |  |  |  |  |  |  |  |  |
|  |  |  |  |  |  |  |  |  |
|  |  |  |  |  |  |  |  |  |

| CARDIO: | TIME | DISTANCE | PACE | HR |
|---|---|---|---|---|
|  |  |  |  |  |
|  |  |  |  |  |
|  |  |  |  |  |
|  |  |  |  |  |

| SUPPLEMENTS & VITAMINS | SERVINGS | QUANTITY |
|---|---|---|
|  |  |  |
|  |  |  |
|  |  |  |
|  |  |  |
|  |  |  |

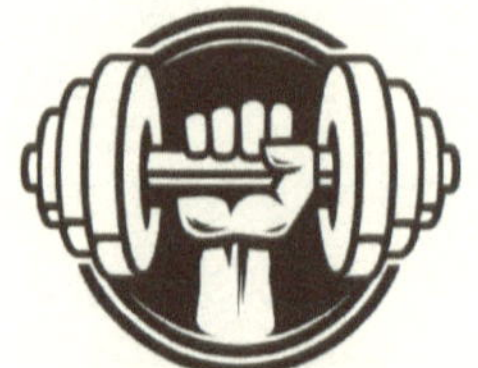

NAME:______________________________

DATE:______________________________

TIME START:______________________________

TIME END:______________________________

| WARM-UP | TIME | NOTES |
|---|---|---|
|  |  |  |
|  |  |  |
|  |  |  |
|  |  |  |

| EXERCISE: | SET 1 | | SET 2 | | SET 3 | | SET 4 | |
|---|---|---|---|---|---|---|---|---|
|  | REPS | WEIGHT | REPS | WEIGHT | REPS | WEIGHT | REPS | WEIGHT |
|  |  |  |  |  |  |  |  |  |
|  |  |  |  |  |  |  |  |  |
|  |  |  |  |  |  |  |  |  |
|  |  |  |  |  |  |  |  |  |
|  |  |  |  |  |  |  |  |  |
|  |  |  |  |  |  |  |  |  |
|  |  |  |  |  |  |  |  |  |
|  |  |  |  |  |  |  |  |  |
|  |  |  |  |  |  |  |  |  |
|  |  |  |  |  |  |  |  |  |
|  |  |  |  |  |  |  |  |  |

| CARDIO: | TIME | DISTANCE | PACE | HR |
|---|---|---|---|---|
|  |  |  |  |  |
|  |  |  |  |  |
|  |  |  |  |  |
|  |  |  |  |  |

| SUPPLEMENTS & VITAMINS | SERVINGS | QUANTITY |
|---|---|---|
|  |  |  |
|  |  |  |
|  |  |  |
|  |  |  |

NAME:_____________________

DATE:_____________________

TIME START:_____________________

TIME END:_____________________

| WARM-UP | TIME | NOTES |
|---|---|---|
|  |  |  |
|  |  |  |
|  |  |  |
|  |  |  |

| EXERCISE: | SET 1 | | SET 2 | | SET 3 | | SET 4 | |
|---|---|---|---|---|---|---|---|---|
|  | REPS | WEIGHT | REPS | WEIGHT | REPS | WEIGHT | REPS | WEIGHT |
|  |  |  |  |  |  |  |  |  |
|  |  |  |  |  |  |  |  |  |
|  |  |  |  |  |  |  |  |  |
|  |  |  |  |  |  |  |  |  |
|  |  |  |  |  |  |  |  |  |
|  |  |  |  |  |  |  |  |  |
|  |  |  |  |  |  |  |  |  |
|  |  |  |  |  |  |  |  |  |
|  |  |  |  |  |  |  |  |  |
|  |  |  |  |  |  |  |  |  |
|  |  |  |  |  |  |  |  |  |

| CARDIO: | TIME | DISTANCE | PACE | HR |
|---|---|---|---|---|
|  |  |  |  |  |
|  |  |  |  |  |
|  |  |  |  |  |

| SUPPLEMENTS & VITAMINS | SERVINGS | QUANTITY |
|---|---|---|
|  |  |  |
|  |  |  |
|  |  |  |
|  |  |  |

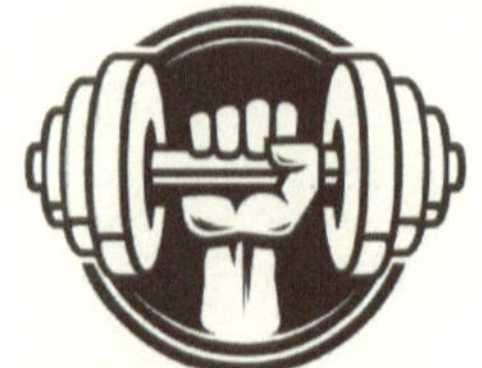

**NAME:**_______________________

**DATE:**_______________________

**TIME START:**_______________________

**TIME END:**_______________________

| WARM-UP | TIME | NOTES |
|---|---|---|
|  |  |  |
|  |  |  |
|  |  |  |
|  |  |  |

| EXERCISE: | SET 1 | | SET 2 | | SET 3 | | SET 4 | |
|---|---|---|---|---|---|---|---|---|
|  | REPS | WEIGHT | REPS | WEIGHT | REPS | WEIGHT | REPS | WEIGHT |
|  |  |  |  |  |  |  |  |  |
|  |  |  |  |  |  |  |  |  |
|  |  |  |  |  |  |  |  |  |
|  |  |  |  |  |  |  |  |  |
|  |  |  |  |  |  |  |  |  |
|  |  |  |  |  |  |  |  |  |
|  |  |  |  |  |  |  |  |  |
|  |  |  |  |  |  |  |  |  |
|  |  |  |  |  |  |  |  |  |
|  |  |  |  |  |  |  |  |  |
|  |  |  |  |  |  |  |  |  |

| CARDIO: | TIME | DISTANCE | PACE | HR |
|---|---|---|---|---|
|  |  |  |  |  |
|  |  |  |  |  |
|  |  |  |  |  |
|  |  |  |  |  |

| SUPPLEMENTS & VITAMINS | SERVINGS | QUANTITY |
|---|---|---|
|  |  |  |
|  |  |  |
|  |  |  |
|  |  |  |
|  |  |  |

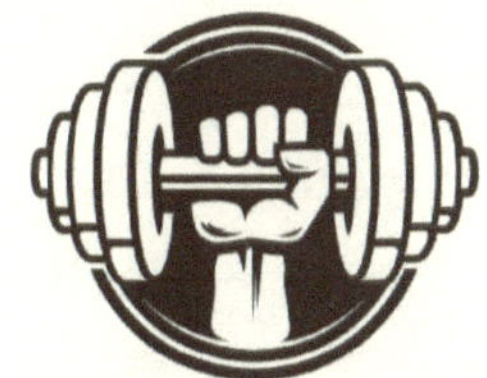

NAME:_______________________

DATE:_______________________

TIME START:_______________________

TIME END:_______________________

| WARM-UP | TIME | NOTES |
|---|---|---|
|  |  |  |
|  |  |  |
|  |  |  |
|  |  |  |

| EXERCISE: | SET 1 | | SET 2 | | SET 3 | | SET 4 | |
|---|---|---|---|---|---|---|---|---|
|  | REPS | WEIGHT | REPS | WEIGHT | REPS | WEIGHT | REPS | WEIGHT |
|  |  |  |  |  |  |  |  |  |
|  |  |  |  |  |  |  |  |  |
|  |  |  |  |  |  |  |  |  |
|  |  |  |  |  |  |  |  |  |
|  |  |  |  |  |  |  |  |  |
|  |  |  |  |  |  |  |  |  |
|  |  |  |  |  |  |  |  |  |
|  |  |  |  |  |  |  |  |  |
|  |  |  |  |  |  |  |  |  |
|  |  |  |  |  |  |  |  |  |
|  |  |  |  |  |  |  |  |  |

| CARDIO: | TIME | DISTANCE | PACE | HR |
|---|---|---|---|---|
|  |  |  |  |  |
|  |  |  |  |  |
|  |  |  |  |  |
|  |  |  |  |  |

| SUPPLEMENTS & VITAMINS | SERVINGS | QUANTITY |
|---|---|---|
|  |  |  |
|  |  |  |
|  |  |  |
|  |  |  |
|  |  |  |

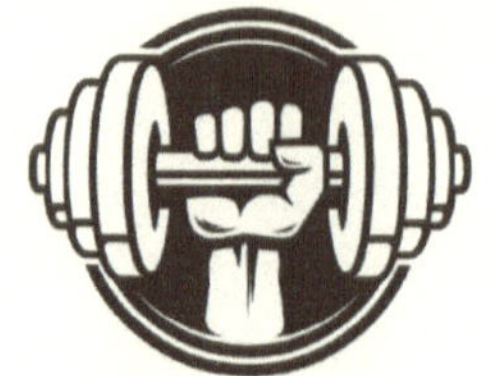

NAME:_______________________

DATE:_______________________

TIME START:_______________________

TIME END:_______________________

| WARM-UP | TIME | NOTES |
|---|---|---|
|  |  |  |
|  |  |  |
|  |  |  |
|  |  |  |

| EXERCISE: | SET 1 | | SET 2 | | SET 3 | | SET 4 | |
|---|---|---|---|---|---|---|---|---|
|  | REPS | WEIGHT | REPS | WEIGHT | REPS | WEIGHT | REPS | WEIGHT |
|  |  |  |  |  |  |  |  |  |
|  |  |  |  |  |  |  |  |  |
|  |  |  |  |  |  |  |  |  |
|  |  |  |  |  |  |  |  |  |
|  |  |  |  |  |  |  |  |  |
|  |  |  |  |  |  |  |  |  |
|  |  |  |  |  |  |  |  |  |
|  |  |  |  |  |  |  |  |  |
|  |  |  |  |  |  |  |  |  |
|  |  |  |  |  |  |  |  |  |
|  |  |  |  |  |  |  |  |  |
|  |  |  |  |  |  |  |  |  |

| CARDIO: | TIME | DISTANCE | PACE | HR |
|---|---|---|---|---|
|  |  |  |  |  |
|  |  |  |  |  |
|  |  |  |  |  |
|  |  |  |  |  |

| SUPPLEMENTS & VITAMINS | SERVINGS | QUANTITY |
|---|---|---|
|  |  |  |
|  |  |  |
|  |  |  |
|  |  |  |
|  |  |  |

NAME: ___________________

DATE: ___________________

TIME START: ___________________

TIME END: ___________________

| WARM-UP | TIME | NOTES |
|---|---|---|
| | | |
| | | |
| | | |
| | | |

| EXERCISE: | SET 1 | | SET 2 | | SET 3 | | SET 4 | |
|---|---|---|---|---|---|---|---|---|
| | REPS | WEIGHT | REPS | WEIGHT | REPS | WEIGHT | REPS | WEIGHT |
| | | | | | | | | |
| | | | | | | | | |
| | | | | | | | | |
| | | | | | | | | |
| | | | | | | | | |
| | | | | | | | | |
| | | | | | | | | |
| | | | | | | | | |
| | | | | | | | | |
| | | | | | | | | |
| | | | | | | | | |

| CARDIO: | TIME | DISTANCE | PACE | HR |
|---|---|---|---|---|
| | | | | |
| | | | | |
| | | | | |
| | | | | |

| SUPPLEMENTS & VITAMINS | SERVINGS | QUANTITY |
|---|---|---|
| | | |
| | | |
| | | |
| | | |
| | | |

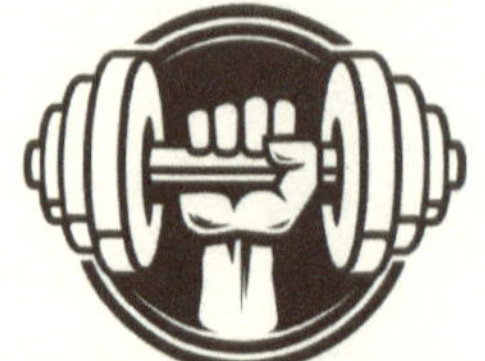

NAME:_______________________________

DATE:_______________________________

TIME START:_______________________________

TIME END:_______________________________

| WARM-UP | TIME | NOTES |
|---|---|---|
|  |  |  |
|  |  |  |
|  |  |  |
|  |  |  |

| EXERCISE: | SET 1 | | SET 2 | | SET 3 | | SET 4 | |
|---|---|---|---|---|---|---|---|---|
|  | REPS | WEIGHT | REPS | WEIGHT | REPS | WEIGHT | REPS | WEIGHT |
|  |  |  |  |  |  |  |  |  |
|  |  |  |  |  |  |  |  |  |
|  |  |  |  |  |  |  |  |  |
|  |  |  |  |  |  |  |  |  |
|  |  |  |  |  |  |  |  |  |
|  |  |  |  |  |  |  |  |  |
|  |  |  |  |  |  |  |  |  |
|  |  |  |  |  |  |  |  |  |
|  |  |  |  |  |  |  |  |  |
|  |  |  |  |  |  |  |  |  |
|  |  |  |  |  |  |  |  |  |
|  |  |  |  |  |  |  |  |  |
|  |  |  |  |  |  |  |  |  |

| CARDIO: | TIME | DISTANCE | PACE | HR |
|---|---|---|---|---|
|  |  |  |  |  |
|  |  |  |  |  |
|  |  |  |  |  |
|  |  |  |  |  |

| SUPPLEMENTS & VITAMINS | SERVINGS | QUANTITY |
|---|---|---|
|  |  |  |
|  |  |  |
|  |  |  |
|  |  |  |
|  |  |  |

NAME: ___________________________

DATE: ___________________________

TIME START: ___________________________

TIME END: ___________________________

| WARM-UP | TIME | NOTES |
|---|---|---|
|  |  |  |
|  |  |  |
|  |  |  |
|  |  |  |

| EXERCISE: | SET 1 | | SET 2 | | SET 3 | | SET 4 | |
|---|---|---|---|---|---|---|---|---|
|  | REPS | WEIGHT | REPS | WEIGHT | REPS | WEIGHT | REPS | WEIGHT |
|  |  |  |  |  |  |  |  |  |
|  |  |  |  |  |  |  |  |  |
|  |  |  |  |  |  |  |  |  |
|  |  |  |  |  |  |  |  |  |
|  |  |  |  |  |  |  |  |  |
|  |  |  |  |  |  |  |  |  |
|  |  |  |  |  |  |  |  |  |
|  |  |  |  |  |  |  |  |  |
|  |  |  |  |  |  |  |  |  |
|  |  |  |  |  |  |  |  |  |

| CARDIO: | TIME | DISTANCE | PACE | HR |
|---|---|---|---|---|
|  |  |  |  |  |
|  |  |  |  |  |
|  |  |  |  |  |
|  |  |  |  |  |

| SUPPLEMENTS & VITAMINS | SERVINGS | QUANTITY |
|---|---|---|
|  |  |  |
|  |  |  |
|  |  |  |
|  |  |  |
|  |  |  |

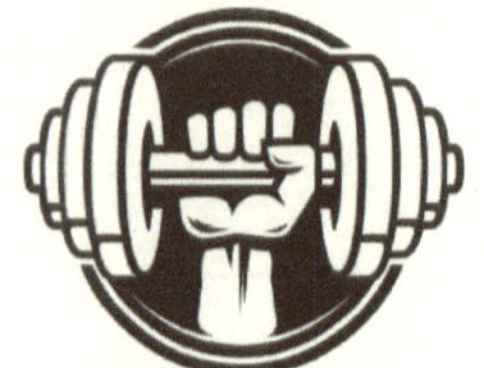

NAME: ___________________________

DATE: ___________________________

TIME START: ___________________________

TIME END: ___________________________

| WARM-UP | TIME | NOTES |
|---|---|---|
|  |  |  |
|  |  |  |
|  |  |  |
|  |  |  |

| EXERCISE: | SET 1 | | SET 2 | | SET 3 | | SET 4 | |
|---|---|---|---|---|---|---|---|---|
|  | REPS | WEIGHT | REPS | WEIGHT | REPS | WEIGHT | REPS | WEIGHT |
|  |  |  |  |  |  |  |  |  |
|  |  |  |  |  |  |  |  |  |
|  |  |  |  |  |  |  |  |  |
|  |  |  |  |  |  |  |  |  |
|  |  |  |  |  |  |  |  |  |
|  |  |  |  |  |  |  |  |  |
|  |  |  |  |  |  |  |  |  |
|  |  |  |  |  |  |  |  |  |
|  |  |  |  |  |  |  |  |  |
|  |  |  |  |  |  |  |  |  |

| CARDIO: | TIME | DISTANCE | PACE | HR |
|---|---|---|---|---|
|  |  |  |  |  |
|  |  |  |  |  |
|  |  |  |  |  |
|  |  |  |  |  |

| SUPPLEMENTS & VITAMINS | SERVINGS | QUANTITY |
|---|---|---|
|  |  |  |
|  |  |  |
|  |  |  |
|  |  |  |

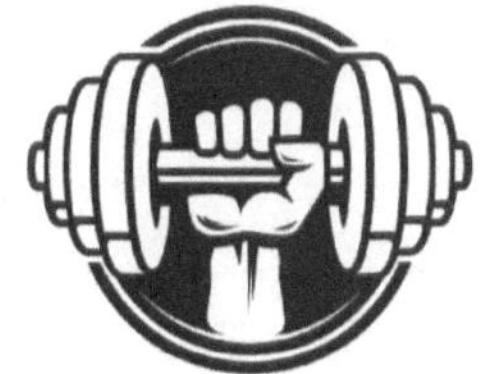

NAME:

DATE:

TIME START:

TIME END:

| WARM-UP | TIME | NOTES |
|---|---|---|
|  |  |  |
|  |  |  |
|  |  |  |

| EXERCISE: | SET 1 | | SET 2 | | SET 3 | | SET 4 | |
|---|---|---|---|---|---|---|---|---|
|  | REPS | WEIGHT | REPS | WEIGHT | REPS | WEIGHT | REPS | WEIGHT |
|  |  |  |  |  |  |  |  |  |
|  |  |  |  |  |  |  |  |  |
|  |  |  |  |  |  |  |  |  |
|  |  |  |  |  |  |  |  |  |
|  |  |  |  |  |  |  |  |  |
|  |  |  |  |  |  |  |  |  |
|  |  |  |  |  |  |  |  |  |
|  |  |  |  |  |  |  |  |  |
|  |  |  |  |  |  |  |  |  |
|  |  |  |  |  |  |  |  |  |

| CARDIO: | TIME | DISTANCE | PACE | HR |
|---|---|---|---|---|
|  |  |  |  |  |
|  |  |  |  |  |
|  |  |  |  |  |

| SUPPLEMENTS & VITAMINS | SERVINGS | QUANTITY |
|---|---|---|
|  |  |  |
|  |  |  |
|  |  |  |

NAME:________________

DATE:________________

TIME START:________________

TIME END:________________

| WARM-UP | TIME | NOTES |
|---|---|---|
|  |  |  |
|  |  |  |
|  |  |  |
|  |  |  |

| EXERCISE: | SET 1 | | SET 2 | | SET 3 | | SET 4 | |
|---|---|---|---|---|---|---|---|---|
|  | REPS | WEIGHT | REPS | WEIGHT | REPS | WEIGHT | REPS | WEIGHT |
|  |  |  |  |  |  |  |  |  |
|  |  |  |  |  |  |  |  |  |
|  |  |  |  |  |  |  |  |  |
|  |  |  |  |  |  |  |  |  |
|  |  |  |  |  |  |  |  |  |
|  |  |  |  |  |  |  |  |  |
|  |  |  |  |  |  |  |  |  |
|  |  |  |  |  |  |  |  |  |
|  |  |  |  |  |  |  |  |  |
|  |  |  |  |  |  |  |  |  |
|  |  |  |  |  |  |  |  |  |
|  |  |  |  |  |  |  |  |  |

| CARDIO: | TIME | DISTANCE | PACE | HR |
|---|---|---|---|---|
|  |  |  |  |  |
|  |  |  |  |  |
|  |  |  |  |  |
|  |  |  |  |  |

| SUPPLEMENTS & VITAMINS | SERVINGS | QUANTITY |
|---|---|---|
|  |  |  |
|  |  |  |
|  |  |  |
|  |  |  |
|  |  |  |

| NAME: | |
| DATE: | |
| TIME START: | |
| TIME END: | |

| WARM-UP | TIME | NOTES |
|---|---|---|
| | | |
| | | |
| | | |
| | | |

| EXERCISE: | SET 1 | | SET 2 | | SET 3 | | SET 4 | |
|---|---|---|---|---|---|---|---|---|
| | REPS | WEIGHT | REPS | WEIGHT | REPS | WEIGHT | REPS | WEIGHT |
| | | | | | | | | |
| | | | | | | | | |
| | | | | | | | | |
| | | | | | | | | |
| | | | | | | | | |
| | | | | | | | | |
| | | | | | | | | |
| | | | | | | | | |
| | | | | | | | | |
| | | | | | | | | |
| | | | | | | | | |
| | | | | | | | | |

| CARDIO: | TIME | DISTANCE | PACE | HR |
|---|---|---|---|---|
| | | | | |
| | | | | |
| | | | | |
| | | | | |

| SUPPLEMENTS & VITAMINS | SERVINGS | QUANTITY |
|---|---|---|
| | | |
| | | |
| | | |
| | | |
| | | |

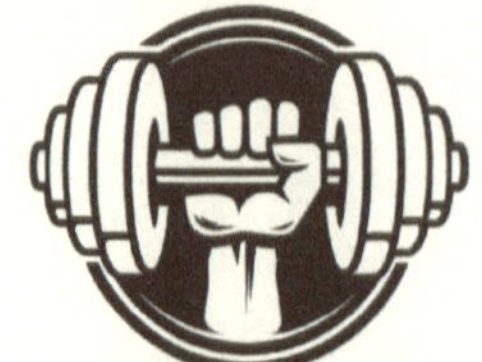

NAME: _______________________

DATE: _______________________

TIME START: _______________________

TIME END: _______________________

| WARM-UP | TIME | NOTES |
|---|---|---|
|  |  |  |
|  |  |  |
|  |  |  |
|  |  |  |

| EXERCISE: | SET 1 | | SET 2 | | SET 3 | | SET 4 | |
|---|---|---|---|---|---|---|---|---|
|  | REPS | WEIGHT | REPS | WEIGHT | REPS | WEIGHT | REPS | WEIGHT |
|  |  |  |  |  |  |  |  |  |
|  |  |  |  |  |  |  |  |  |
|  |  |  |  |  |  |  |  |  |
|  |  |  |  |  |  |  |  |  |
|  |  |  |  |  |  |  |  |  |
|  |  |  |  |  |  |  |  |  |
|  |  |  |  |  |  |  |  |  |
|  |  |  |  |  |  |  |  |  |
|  |  |  |  |  |  |  |  |  |
|  |  |  |  |  |  |  |  |  |
|  |  |  |  |  |  |  |  |  |

| CARDIO: | TIME | DISTANCE | PACE | HR |
|---|---|---|---|---|
|  |  |  |  |  |
|  |  |  |  |  |
|  |  |  |  |  |
|  |  |  |  |  |

| SUPPLEMENTS & VITAMINS | SERVINGS | QUANTITY |
|---|---|---|
|  |  |  |
|  |  |  |
|  |  |  |
|  |  |  |

NAME:

DATE:

TIME START:

TIME END:

| WARM-UP | TIME | NOTES |
|---|---|---|
|  |  |  |
|  |  |  |
|  |  |  |
|  |  |  |

| EXERCISE: | SET 1 | | SET 2 | | SET 3 | | SET 4 | |
|---|---|---|---|---|---|---|---|---|
|  | REPS | WEIGHT | REPS | WEIGHT | REPS | WEIGHT | REPS | WEIGHT |
|  |  |  |  |  |  |  |  |  |
|  |  |  |  |  |  |  |  |  |
|  |  |  |  |  |  |  |  |  |
|  |  |  |  |  |  |  |  |  |
|  |  |  |  |  |  |  |  |  |
|  |  |  |  |  |  |  |  |  |
|  |  |  |  |  |  |  |  |  |
|  |  |  |  |  |  |  |  |  |
|  |  |  |  |  |  |  |  |  |
|  |  |  |  |  |  |  |  |  |

| CARDIO: | TIME | DISTANCE | PACE | HR |
|---|---|---|---|---|
|  |  |  |  |  |
|  |  |  |  |  |
|  |  |  |  |  |
|  |  |  |  |  |

| SUPPLEMENTS & VITAMINS | SERVINGS | QUANTITY |
|---|---|---|
|  |  |  |
|  |  |  |
|  |  |  |
|  |  |  |
|  |  |  |

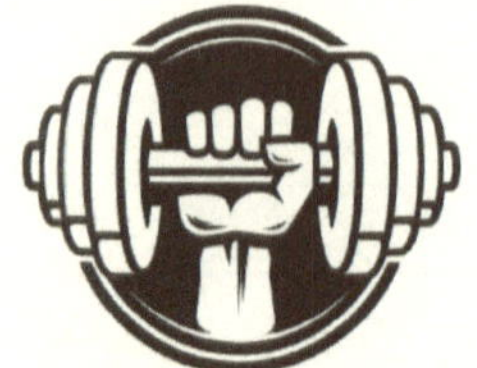

NAME:

DATE:

TIME START:

TIME END:

| WARM-UP | TIME | NOTES |
|---------|------|-------|
|  |  |  |
|  |  |  |
|  |  |  |
|  |  |  |

| EXERCISE: | SET 1 | | SET 2 | | SET 3 | | SET 4 | |
|-----------|-------|--------|-------|--------|-------|--------|-------|--------|
|  | REPS | WEIGHT | REPS | WEIGHT | REPS | WEIGHT | REPS | WEIGHT |
|  |  |  |  |  |  |  |  |  |
|  |  |  |  |  |  |  |  |  |
|  |  |  |  |  |  |  |  |  |
|  |  |  |  |  |  |  |  |  |
|  |  |  |  |  |  |  |  |  |
|  |  |  |  |  |  |  |  |  |
|  |  |  |  |  |  |  |  |  |
|  |  |  |  |  |  |  |  |  |
|  |  |  |  |  |  |  |  |  |
|  |  |  |  |  |  |  |  |  |
|  |  |  |  |  |  |  |  |  |
|  |  |  |  |  |  |  |  |  |

| CARDIO: | TIME | DISTANCE | PACE | HR |
|---------|------|----------|------|-----|
|  |  |  |  |  |
|  |  |  |  |  |
|  |  |  |  |  |
|  |  |  |  |  |

| SUPPLEMENTS & VITAMINS | SERVINGS | QUANTITY |
|------------------------|----------|----------|
|  |  |  |
|  |  |  |
|  |  |  |
|  |  |  |
|  |  |  |

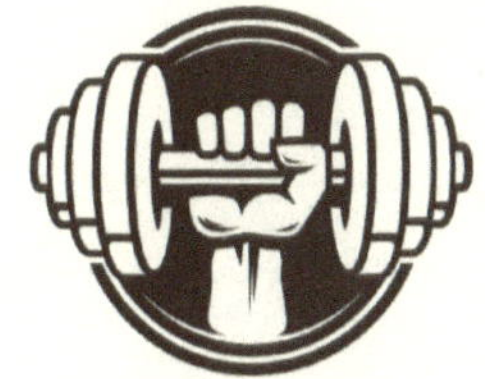

NAME:_______________________

DATE:_______________________

TIME START:_______________________

TIME END:_______________________

| WARM-UP | TIME | NOTES |
|---|---|---|
|  |  |  |
|  |  |  |
|  |  |  |
|  |  |  |

| EXERCISE: | SET 1 | | SET 2 | | SET 3 | | SET 4 | |
|---|---|---|---|---|---|---|---|---|
|  | REPS | WEIGHT | REPS | WEIGHT | REPS | WEIGHT | REPS | WEIGHT |
|  |  |  |  |  |  |  |  |  |
|  |  |  |  |  |  |  |  |  |
|  |  |  |  |  |  |  |  |  |
|  |  |  |  |  |  |  |  |  |
|  |  |  |  |  |  |  |  |  |
|  |  |  |  |  |  |  |  |  |
|  |  |  |  |  |  |  |  |  |
|  |  |  |  |  |  |  |  |  |
|  |  |  |  |  |  |  |  |  |
|  |  |  |  |  |  |  |  |  |
|  |  |  |  |  |  |  |  |  |

| CARDIO: | TIME | DISTANCE | PACE | HR |
|---|---|---|---|---|
|  |  |  |  |  |
|  |  |  |  |  |
|  |  |  |  |  |
|  |  |  |  |  |

| SUPPLEMENTS & VITAMINS | SERVINGS | QUANTITY |
|---|---|---|
|  |  |  |
|  |  |  |
|  |  |  |
|  |  |  |
|  |  |  |

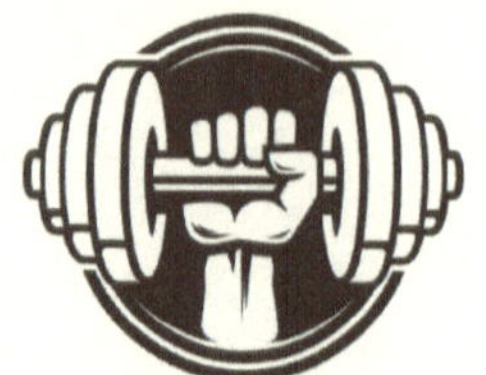

**NAME:** _______________________

**DATE:** _______________________

**TIME START:** _______________________

**TIME END:** _______________________

| WARM-UP | TIME | NOTES |
|---|---|---|
|  |  |  |
|  |  |  |
|  |  |  |

| EXERCISE: | SET 1 | | SET 2 | | SET 3 | | SET 4 | |
|---|---|---|---|---|---|---|---|---|
|  | REPS | WEIGHT | REPS | WEIGHT | REPS | WEIGHT | REPS | WEIGHT |
|  |  |  |  |  |  |  |  |  |
|  |  |  |  |  |  |  |  |  |
|  |  |  |  |  |  |  |  |  |
|  |  |  |  |  |  |  |  |  |
|  |  |  |  |  |  |  |  |  |
|  |  |  |  |  |  |  |  |  |
|  |  |  |  |  |  |  |  |  |
|  |  |  |  |  |  |  |  |  |
|  |  |  |  |  |  |  |  |  |

| CARDIO: | TIME | DISTANCE | PACE | HR |
|---|---|---|---|---|
|  |  |  |  |  |
|  |  |  |  |  |
|  |  |  |  |  |

| SUPPLEMENTS & VITAMINS | SERVINGS | QUANTITY |
|---|---|---|
|  |  |  |
|  |  |  |
|  |  |  |
|  |  |  |

| NAME: | |
|---|---|
| DATE: | |
| TIME START: | |
| TIME END: | |

| WARM-UP | TIME | NOTES |
|---|---|---|
| | | |
| | | |
| | | |
| | | |

| EXERCISE: | SET 1 | | SET 2 | | SET 3 | | SET 4 | |
|---|---|---|---|---|---|---|---|---|
| | REPS | WEIGHT | REPS | WEIGHT | REPS | WEIGHT | REPS | WEIGHT |
| | | | | | | | | |
| | | | | | | | | |
| | | | | | | | | |
| | | | | | | | | |
| | | | | | | | | |
| | | | | | | | | |
| | | | | | | | | |
| | | | | | | | | |
| | | | | | | | | |
| | | | | | | | | |

| CARDIO: | TIME | DISTANCE | PACE | HR |
|---|---|---|---|---|
| | | | | |
| | | | | |
| | | | | |
| | | | | |

| SUPPLEMENTS & VITAMINS | SERVINGS | QUANTITY |
|---|---|---|
| | | |
| | | |
| | | |
| | | |
| | | |

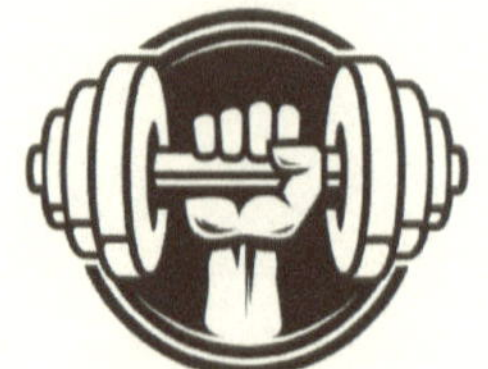

NAME:

DATE:

TIME START:

TIME END:

| WARM-UP | TIME | NOTES |
|---|---|---|
|  |  |  |
|  |  |  |
|  |  |  |
|  |  |  |

| EXERCISE: | SET 1 | | SET 2 | | SET 3 | | SET 4 | |
|---|---|---|---|---|---|---|---|---|
|  | REPS | WEIGHT | REPS | WEIGHT | REPS | WEIGHT | REPS | WEIGHT |
|  |  |  |  |  |  |  |  |  |
|  |  |  |  |  |  |  |  |  |
|  |  |  |  |  |  |  |  |  |
|  |  |  |  |  |  |  |  |  |
|  |  |  |  |  |  |  |  |  |
|  |  |  |  |  |  |  |  |  |
|  |  |  |  |  |  |  |  |  |
|  |  |  |  |  |  |  |  |  |
|  |  |  |  |  |  |  |  |  |
|  |  |  |  |  |  |  |  |  |
|  |  |  |  |  |  |  |  |  |
|  |  |  |  |  |  |  |  |  |

| CARDIO: | TIME | DISTANCE | PACE | HR |
|---|---|---|---|---|
|  |  |  |  |  |
|  |  |  |  |  |
|  |  |  |  |  |
|  |  |  |  |  |

| SUPPLEMENTS & VITAMINS | SERVINGS | QUANTITY |
|---|---|---|
|  |  |  |
|  |  |  |
|  |  |  |
|  |  |  |
|  |  |  |

NAME:_______________________________

DATE:_______________________________

TIME START:_______________________________

TIME END:_______________________________

| WARM-UP | TIME | NOTES |
|---|---|---|
|  |  |  |
|  |  |  |
|  |  |  |
|  |  |  |

| EXERCISE: | SET 1 | | SET 2 | | SET 3 | | SET 4 | |
|---|---|---|---|---|---|---|---|---|
|  | REPS | WEIGHT | REPS | WEIGHT | REPS | WEIGHT | REPS | WEIGHT |
|  |  |  |  |  |  |  |  |  |
|  |  |  |  |  |  |  |  |  |
|  |  |  |  |  |  |  |  |  |
|  |  |  |  |  |  |  |  |  |
|  |  |  |  |  |  |  |  |  |
|  |  |  |  |  |  |  |  |  |
|  |  |  |  |  |  |  |  |  |
|  |  |  |  |  |  |  |  |  |
|  |  |  |  |  |  |  |  |  |
|  |  |  |  |  |  |  |  |  |
|  |  |  |  |  |  |  |  |  |

| CARDIO: | TIME | DISTANCE | PACE | HR |
|---|---|---|---|---|
|  |  |  |  |  |
|  |  |  |  |  |
|  |  |  |  |  |
|  |  |  |  |  |

| SUPPLEMENTS & VITAMINS | SERVINGS | QUANTITY |
|---|---|---|
|  |  |  |
|  |  |  |
|  |  |  |
|  |  |  |
|  |  |  |

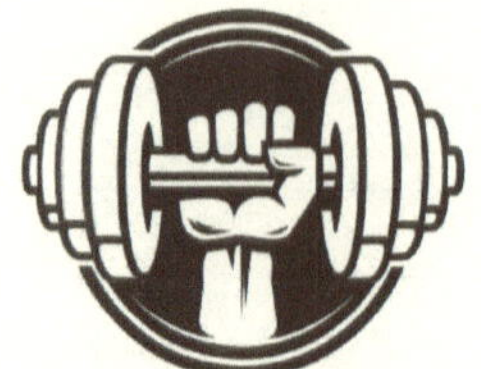

NAME:

DATE:

TIME START:

TIME END:

| WARM-UP | TIME | NOTES |
|---|---|---|
|  |  |  |
|  |  |  |
|  |  |  |
|  |  |  |

| EXERCISE: | SET 1 | | SET 2 | | SET 3 | | SET 4 | |
|---|---|---|---|---|---|---|---|---|
|  | REPS | WEIGHT | REPS | WEIGHT | REPS | WEIGHT | REPS | WEIGHT |
|  |  |  |  |  |  |  |  |  |
|  |  |  |  |  |  |  |  |  |
|  |  |  |  |  |  |  |  |  |
|  |  |  |  |  |  |  |  |  |
|  |  |  |  |  |  |  |  |  |
|  |  |  |  |  |  |  |  |  |
|  |  |  |  |  |  |  |  |  |
|  |  |  |  |  |  |  |  |  |
|  |  |  |  |  |  |  |  |  |
|  |  |  |  |  |  |  |  |  |
|  |  |  |  |  |  |  |  |  |
|  |  |  |  |  |  |  |  |  |

| CARDIO: | TIME | DISTANCE | PACE | HR |
|---|---|---|---|---|
|  |  |  |  |  |
|  |  |  |  |  |
|  |  |  |  |  |
|  |  |  |  |  |

| SUPPLEMENTS & VITAMINS | SERVINGS | QUANTITY |
|---|---|---|
|  |  |  |
|  |  |  |
|  |  |  |
|  |  |  |

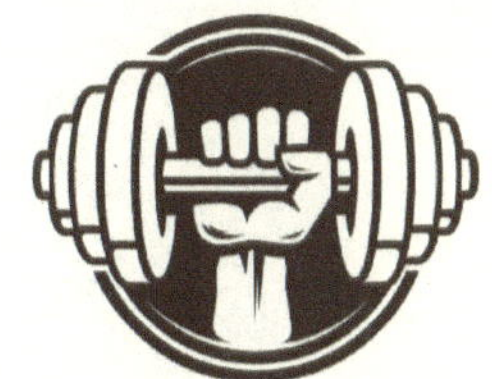

NAME:

DATE:

TIME START:

TIME END:

| WARM-UP | TIME | NOTES |
|---|---|---|
|  |  |  |
|  |  |  |
|  |  |  |
|  |  |  |

| EXERCISE: | SET 1 | | SET 2 | | SET 3 | | SET 4 | |
|---|---|---|---|---|---|---|---|---|
|  | REPS | WEIGHT | REPS | WEIGHT | REPS | WEIGHT | REPS | WEIGHT |
|  |  |  |  |  |  |  |  |  |
|  |  |  |  |  |  |  |  |  |
|  |  |  |  |  |  |  |  |  |
|  |  |  |  |  |  |  |  |  |
|  |  |  |  |  |  |  |  |  |
|  |  |  |  |  |  |  |  |  |
|  |  |  |  |  |  |  |  |  |
|  |  |  |  |  |  |  |  |  |
|  |  |  |  |  |  |  |  |  |
|  |  |  |  |  |  |  |  |  |
|  |  |  |  |  |  |  |  |  |

| CARDIO: | TIME | DISTANCE | PACE | HR |
|---|---|---|---|---|
|  |  |  |  |  |
|  |  |  |  |  |
|  |  |  |  |  |
|  |  |  |  |  |

| SUPPLEMENTS & VITAMINS | SERVINGS | QUANTITY |
|---|---|---|
|  |  |  |
|  |  |  |
|  |  |  |
|  |  |  |
|  |  |  |

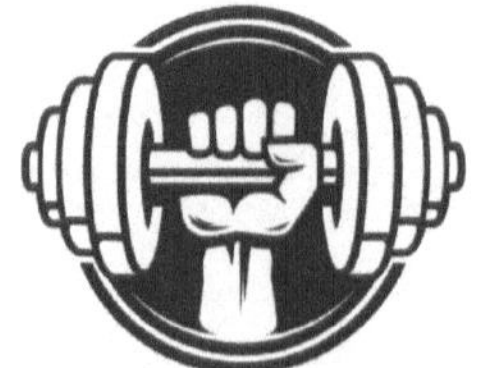

NAME:_______________________

DATE:_______________________

TIME START:_______________________

TIME END:_______________________

| WARM-UP | TIME | NOTES |
|---|---|---|
|  |  |  |
|  |  |  |
|  |  |  |
|  |  |  |

| EXERCISE: | SET 1 | | SET 2 | | SET 3 | | SET 4 | |
|---|---|---|---|---|---|---|---|---|
|  | REPS | WEIGHT | REPS | WEIGHT | REPS | WEIGHT | REPS | WEIGHT |
|  |  |  |  |  |  |  |  |  |
|  |  |  |  |  |  |  |  |  |
|  |  |  |  |  |  |  |  |  |
|  |  |  |  |  |  |  |  |  |
|  |  |  |  |  |  |  |  |  |
|  |  |  |  |  |  |  |  |  |
|  |  |  |  |  |  |  |  |  |
|  |  |  |  |  |  |  |  |  |
|  |  |  |  |  |  |  |  |  |
|  |  |  |  |  |  |  |  |  |
|  |  |  |  |  |  |  |  |  |
|  |  |  |  |  |  |  |  |  |

| CARDIO: | TIME | DISTANCE | PACE | HR |
|---|---|---|---|---|
|  |  |  |  |  |
|  |  |  |  |  |
|  |  |  |  |  |
|  |  |  |  |  |

| SUPPLEMENTS & VITAMINS | SERVINGS | QUANTITY |
|---|---|---|
|  |  |  |
|  |  |  |
|  |  |  |
|  |  |  |

NAME:_______________________________________

DATE:_______________________________________

TIME START:_________________________________

TIME END:___________________________________

| WARM-UP | TIME | NOTES |
|---|---|---|
|  |  |  |
|  |  |  |
|  |  |  |
|  |  |  |

| EXERCISE: | SET 1 | | SET 2 | | SET 3 | | SET 4 | |
|---|---|---|---|---|---|---|---|---|
|  | REPS | WEIGHT | REPS | WEIGHT | REPS | WEIGHT | REPS | WEIGHT |
|  |  |  |  |  |  |  |  |  |
|  |  |  |  |  |  |  |  |  |
|  |  |  |  |  |  |  |  |  |
|  |  |  |  |  |  |  |  |  |
|  |  |  |  |  |  |  |  |  |
|  |  |  |  |  |  |  |  |  |
|  |  |  |  |  |  |  |  |  |
|  |  |  |  |  |  |  |  |  |
|  |  |  |  |  |  |  |  |  |
|  |  |  |  |  |  |  |  |  |
|  |  |  |  |  |  |  |  |  |

| CARDIO: | TIME | DISTANCE | PACE | HR |
|---|---|---|---|---|
|  |  |  |  |  |
|  |  |  |  |  |
|  |  |  |  |  |
|  |  |  |  |  |

| SUPPLEMENTS & VITAMINS | SERVINGS | QUANTITY |
|---|---|---|
|  |  |  |
|  |  |  |
|  |  |  |
|  |  |  |
|  |  |  |

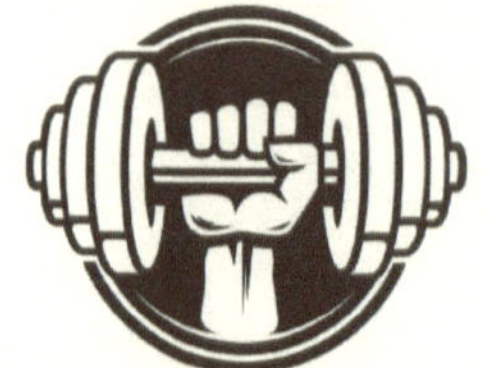

NAME:

DATE:

TIME START:

TIME END:

| WARM-UP | TIME | NOTES |
|---|---|---|
|  |  |  |
|  |  |  |
|  |  |  |
|  |  |  |

| EXERCISE: | SET 1 | | SET 2 | | SET 3 | | SET 4 | |
|---|---|---|---|---|---|---|---|---|
|  | REPS | WEIGHT | REPS | WEIGHT | REPS | WEIGHT | REPS | WEIGHT |
|  |  |  |  |  |  |  |  |  |
|  |  |  |  |  |  |  |  |  |
|  |  |  |  |  |  |  |  |  |
|  |  |  |  |  |  |  |  |  |
|  |  |  |  |  |  |  |  |  |
|  |  |  |  |  |  |  |  |  |
|  |  |  |  |  |  |  |  |  |
|  |  |  |  |  |  |  |  |  |
|  |  |  |  |  |  |  |  |  |
|  |  |  |  |  |  |  |  |  |
|  |  |  |  |  |  |  |  |  |
|  |  |  |  |  |  |  |  |  |

| CARDIO: | TIME | DISTANCE | PACE | HR |
|---|---|---|---|---|
|  |  |  |  |  |
|  |  |  |  |  |
|  |  |  |  |  |
|  |  |  |  |  |

| SUPPLEMENTS & VITAMINS | SERVINGS | QUANTITY |
|---|---|---|
|  |  |  |
|  |  |  |
|  |  |  |
|  |  |  |